The Mental Health Effects of Informal Caregiving:

Emerging Research and Opportunities

Debra Gavin Ware
Argosy University, USA

Tarnue Johnson
Argosy University, USA & Kirkwood Community College, USA

A volume in the Advances in Psychology, Mental Health, and Behavioral Studies (APMHBS) Book Series

IGI Global
DISSEMINATOR OF KNOWLEDGE

Published in the United States of America by
IGI Global
Medical Information Science Reference (an imprint of IGI Global)
701 E. Chocolate Avenue
Hershey PA, USA 17033
Tel: 717-533-8845
Fax: 717-533-8661
E-mail: cust@igi-global.com
Web site: http://www.igi-global.com

Library of Congress Cataloging-in-Publication Data

Names: Gavin Ware, Debra, 1960- author. | Johnson, Tarnue Carver, author.
Title: The mental health effects of informal caregiving : emerging research and opportunities / by Debra Gavin Ware and Tarnue Johnson.
Description: Hershey PA : Medical Information Science Reference, [2019] | Includes bibliographical references.
Identifiers: LCCN 2018028565| ISBN 9781522574521 (hardcover) | ISBN 9781522574538 (ebook)
Subjects: | MESH: Caregivers--psychology | Home Nursing--psychology | Health Services Research
Classification: LCC RA645.35 | NLM WY 200 | DDC 362.14--dc23 LC record available at https://lccn.loc.gov/2018028565

This book is published in the IGI Global book series Advances in Psychology, Mental Health, and Behavioral Studies (APMHBS) (ISSN: 2475-6660; eISSN: 2475-6679)

British Cataloguing in Publication Data
A Cataloguing in Publication record for this book is available from the British Library.

Advances in Psychology, Mental Health, and Behavioral Studies (APMHBS) Book Series

ISSN:2475-6660
EISSN:2475-6679

Editor-in-Chief: Bryan Christiansen, Global Research Society, LLC, USA & Harish C. Chandan, Argosy University, USA

MISSION

The complexity of the human mind has puzzled researchers and physicians for centuries. While widely studied, the brain still remains largely misunderstood.

The **Advances in Psychology, Mental Health, and Behavioral Studies (APMHBS)** book series presents comprehensive research publications focusing on topics relating to the human psyche, cognition, psychiatric care, mental and developmental disorders, as well as human behavior and interaction. Featuring diverse and innovative research, publications within APMHBS are ideally designed for use by mental health professionals, academicians, researchers, and upper-level students.

COVERAGE

- Human Interaction
- Emotional Health
- Addiction
- Personality Disorders
- Trauma & Stress
- Substance Abuse
- Counseling & Therapy
- Cognition
- Human Behavior
- Anxiety

The Advances in Psychology, Mental Health, and Behavioral Studies (APMHBS) Book Series (ISSN 2475-6660) is published by IGI Global, 701 E. Chocolate Avenue, Hershey, PA 17033-1240, USA, www.igi-global.com. This series is composed of titles available for purchase individually; each title is edited to be contextually exclusive from any other title within the series. For pricing and ordering information please visit http://www.igi-global.com/book-series/advances-psychology-mental-health-behavioral/110200. Postmaster: Send all address changes to above address.

Titles in this Series

For a list of additional titles in this series, please visit:
https://www.igi-global.com/book-series/advances-psychology-mental-health-behavioral/110200

Scientific Concepts Behind Happiness, Kindness, and Empathy in Contemporay Society
Nava R. Silton (Marymount Manhattan College, USA)
Information Science Reference • ©2019 • 321pp • H/C (ISBN: 9781522559184) • US $185.00

Handbook of Research on Psychosocial Perspectives of Human Communication Disorders
Sanjeev Kumar Gupta (All India Institute of Speech and Hearing, India) and Srinivasan Venkatesan (All India Institute of Speech and Hearin, India)
Medical Information Science Reference • ©2018 • 465pp • H/C (ISBN: 9781522549550) • US $275.00

Deconstructing Stigma in Mental Health
Brittany A. Canfield (Southern New Hampshire University, USA) and Holly A. Cunningham (CPES Inc., USA)
Medical Information Science Reference • ©2018 • 307pp • H/C (ISBN: 9781522538080) • US $225.00

Social, Psychological, and Forensic Perspectives on Sexual Abuse
Rejani Thudalikunnil Gopalan (Gujarat Forensic Sciences University, India)
Information Science Reference • ©2018 • 374pp • H/C (ISBN: 9781522539582) • US $195.00

Raising Mental Health Awareness in Higher Education Emerging Research and Opportunities
Melissa Martin (State University of New York at Plattsburgh, USA) Jean Mockry (State University of New York at Plattsburgh, USA) Alison Puliatte (State University of New York at Plattsburgh, USA) Denise A. Simard (State University of New York at Plattsburgh, USA) and Maureen E. Squires (State University of New York at Plattsburgh, USA)
Medical Information Science Reference • ©2018 • 136pp • H/C (ISBN: 9781522537939) • US $175.00

For an entire list of titles in this series, please visit:
https://www.igi-global.com/book-series/advances-psychology-mental-health-behavioral/110200

IGI Global
DISSEMINATOR OF KNOWLEDGE

701 East Chocolate Avenue, Hershey, PA 17033, USA
Tel: 717-533-8845 x100 • Fax: 717-533-8661
E-Mail: cust@igi-global.com • www.igi-global.com

Table of Contents

Preface

INTRODUCTION

This book aims to provide research findings that shed light on the factors that impact the social wellbeing of informal caregivers in a variety of contexts. The rationale that undergirds the publication of this book is explained in Chapter 1 and further made evidence through discussions in subsequent chapters. The various groups, both individuals and institutions, that can benefit from this publication are mentioned in Chapter 1. The book has five chapters that include discussions of research design, methodology, presentation and discussion of the research findings as well as a postscript (Chapter 5). The postscript aims to provide a reflective autobiographical account of Dr. Debra Gavin Ware's experience of being an informal caregiver. Meanwhile, Chapter 1 presents the methodological and conceptual approach, which informed the research design for the study. It is pertinent to reiterate here that the design of this study sought to discern the positive psychological forces that shape subjective wellbeing of informal caregivers.

This research objective prompted the adoption of a mixed methods research. The rationale that undergirds this methodological preference is presented. In addition, advantages of mixed methods approach are elaborated upon. Furthermore, other issues are addressed, including sample size, instrumentation as well as research procedures. This chapter also explains, in much detail, the parameters and boundary conditions that constituted the guiding assumptions, limitations, as well as delimitations of the study. It should be noted that the chapter also explains the essential approach to data analysis, which embodied the adoption of descriptive and probabilistic or inferential statistics.

Chapter 2 posits that based on a careful review of extant literature, the quest to identify the factors that assist caregivers in sustaining or elevating their subjective wellbeing while providing comfort and support to care recipients is critical. In this sense, discussion in this chapter provides a rationale for the design and focus of research reported in this book, which focuses on the positive factors that elevate subjective wellbeing of informal caregivers. Thus, this chapter explores various research findings and theoretical discussion on associations between subjective wellbeing and fundamental characteristics of mental and psychical wellness of those providing care on an informal basis. These include the accentuation of self-efficacy, spirituality and other pertinent psychological and social categories.

It also includes the extent to which an informal caregiver receives support from others to enhance a sense of belonging to community. In addition, it further includes personal resilience of the caregiver as well as opportunities to participate in leisure activities and community involvement. This chapter further provides a discussion of how Lawrence Kohlberg's moral development theory helps to explain the positive self-rating of the role of spiritual beliefs in the lives of informal caregivers. Chapter 5 encapsulates discussion of research findings and their relevant policy conclusions and recommendations.

Chapter 4 reports and discusses the finding that research participants had the perception that their spiritual beliefs were positively influential to their caregiver roles and their subjective wellbeing. It also probes the finding that research participants seemed to rely on their spiritual convictions as the lynchpin in sustaining themselves in their roles as informal caregivers as it related to their subjective wellbeing. Similarly, the chapter discusses that the finding that the vast majority of research participants believed their resilience allowed them to be optimistic about their performance as caregivers. Other relevant research findings are also duly discussed.

Chapter 5 encompasses a reflective autobiographic account of the principal investigator, and co-author Dr. Debra Gavin Ware that plumbs the depths of what it means to be an informal caregiver for a family member or loved one. The chapter traces the researcher's steps as a caregiver for her late mother and the joys of personal fulfillment (positive sense of wellbeing) and occasional travails associated with an individual stepping into this role. The researcher use the variables in the study (subjective wellbeing, self-efficacy, spirituality, social support, resilience, and leisure participation) as lenses to discuss a reflective account of her experiences in the context of her own family. The researchers strongly hope that accounts presented in this book would make an essential contribution to advancing the frontiers of psychological and social policy science. And, given the timely nature of this publication, it is small wonder that such an aspiration will be realized.

Introduction

This book could not have come at a very important time, given the exigencies of the historical moment. Indeed, we as an American society are currently experiencing the explosion of caregiving in a variety of settings, including institutional and informal settings. The increasingly elderly and baby boom population has continued to grow as life expectancy continues to improve among all racial groups, including African Americans, requiring more senior care. In addition, the number of children with special healthcare needs across racial categories has also grown. In fact, it has been estimated that 13.9% of children under age 18 have special healthcare needs.

There are also adults in the middle of the developmental lifespan who find themselves incapacitated for one reason or another and in need of care. Among these population groups could be counted veterans from recent wars from Iraq and Afghanistan who have returned home. These public policy and societal challenges demand new understandings and forms of care both in formal institutional and informal settings. They also demand nuanced and scholarly appreciation of the pertinent social and psychological factors that enhance caregiving, especially as a voluntary endeavor by families and love ones of those incapable of caring for themselves.

This book is an outcome of Dr. Debra Gavin Ware's doctoral dissertation research project—a research effort, which in effect was an extension of the author's lived experiences acquired in the context of providing care to her late mother. Since this critical milestone in the author's life, she has always been seized by the question as to which salient and psychological factors affect the subjective wellbeing of informal caregivers. A further rationale for the study stemmed from the realization that there is a paucity of research surrounding the positive aspects of the caregiving experience. A careful reviewed of prior research revealed that prior studies had properly determined, in various statistical magnitudes, the negative consequences associated with the caregiving experience. Hence, on the basis of these presuppositions, the study was purposely designed to explore the influence of presumed positive psychological factors on caregivers, such as self-efficacy, social support, spirituality, resilience, and leisure participation on the subjective wellbeing of the informal caregiver.

The study also examined the aforementioned factors in terms of their implications for managers in 21st century caregiving organizations. Accordingly, crucial changes were made to the original manuscript to make it suitable for a book project of this nature through the collaborative efforts of both authors. Also, various inputs from double blind reviewers commissioned by IGI Global Publishers were made in the publication process that undoubtedly improved this final product.

Readers would note that of specific concern to the authors was exploring the psychological construct of subjective wellbeing and affects that mediate this construct in the context of informal caregiving activities. The research approach adopted in conducting this study was one of a concurrent mixed methods design. In this context, quantitative as well as qualitative approaches were adopted. Crucially, a sample of 36 African American participants from two local religious organizations who categorized themselves as informal caregivers took part in the study. The quantitative analysis portion of the study involved the application of correlation and regression methods to determine the extent to which the dependent variable (i.e., subjective wellbeing) was influenced by the independent variables (i.e., self-efficacy, social support, spirituality, leisure participation, and resilience).

The results reported in this book showed a statistically significant relationship between each variable and subjective wellbeing, with the exception of resilience. Results of a stepwise regression analysis showed that the number of months an informal caregiver spent providing care was a significant positive predictor of subjective wellbeing. Additionally, results of the qualitative analysis showed that informal caregivers believed all of the independent variables or factors delineated in the study reported here affected their subjective wellbeing.

These caregivers often perceived their responsibilities to the care recipient as an act of love and contended that the aforementioned independent variables were important factors in enhancing their subjective wellbeing in terms of helping them to better manage their caregiving responsibilities. The findings are supported by prior empirical and theoretical studies. The current text also recommends that future empirical inquiry be encouraged to examine the effects of implementing programs and public policies designed to assist informal caregivers and in so doing add to the refinement and contextual efficacy of these policies and programs.

These researchers are convinced that various groups and stakeholders can benefit from this publication. These include scholar practitioners working in higher education and those working as clinical therapists in private practice. Undergraduate and graduate students studying psychology or other behavioral sciences could benefit from reading this publication. Informal caregivers with a professional background in the fields of psychology or other behavioral sciences could also benefit immensely from incorporating the research findings of this book in their analytical frameworks and approaches. Finally, nonprofit organizations and other institutional stakeholders could from research findings reported in this book.

ORGANIZATION OF THE BOOK

This section provides an introductory summary and goes beyond that to conduct an evaluation of the significance of this book in terms of current trends and research results. Chapter 1 reflects critical discussion of the state of research on subjective wellbeing. This chapter posits that the quest to identify factors that assist caregivers in maintaining and elevating their subjective wellbeing while providing nurturing and support to caregivers is critical.

The chapter further states that the design of this study was gear at empirically examining various constructs in ways that fit the essential research problem. The chapter ends with an attempt by the authors to explore the link between Kohlberg's developmental theory and subjective wellbeing. The authors rendered various conjectures concerning the cognitive-developmental implications of some of the factors (i.e., self-efficacy, social support, resilience, spirituality and leisure participation) that tend to elevate or diminish subjective wellbeing of informal caregivers as a result of providing care to love ones.

Meanwhile, Chapter 2 presents the methodological and conceptual framework of the study. This chapter explains that the study relied on the use of a concurrent mixed methods research design, including the sample selection process, sample size, selection of participants, instrument, methodological assumptions, procedures, limitations, data collection methods, and data analysis. Chapter 3 focuses on the presentation of research findings. In effect, chapter three provides the crucial link that exists between the articulation of the research problem, generation of data and the empirical findings discussed in chapter four. Chapter 4 presents discussions of research results in view of extent literature and makes series of policy recommendations for both future research endeavors and policy development. Finally, Chapter 5 presents a reflective account of one of the authors (Dr. Debra Gavin Ware) regarding critical aspects of her experience as an informal caregiver. The aim of this reflective account was to walk readers through some aspects of how the author experienced the interaction of subject wellbeing and the independent variables.

STATEMENT OF THE PROBLEM

There is a paucity of research surrounding the positive aspects of the caregiving experience. To address this issue, the current study was designed to explore the influence of self-efficacy, social support, spirituality, resilience, and leisure participation on the subjective wellbeing of the informal caregiver. Prior research has clearly revealed the negative consequences associated with the role of the informal caregiver. These concerns include, but are not limited to, such issues as emotional episodes, financial stress, ill health, and even an increased risk of mortality experienced by informal caregivers (Cohen, Colantonio, & Vernich, 2002; Haley, LaMonde, Han, Burton, & Schonwetter, 2003; Robinson, 1983). However, these authors content that to further understand the informal caregiver perspective; researchers must begin to examine the positive factors expressed by the caregivers themselves (Cohen et al., 2002). This is the gap in research that the current study was designed to address.

As the positive aspects of caregiving have received so little attention, there are many things about the informal caregiver environment that remain a mystery. A number of authors have explored the effects of positive feelings as they relate to informal caregiving (Allen, 2003; Cohen et al., 2002; Kramer, 1997). The known studies pertaining to the positive aspects of caregiving involved investigations of a variety of operational definitions, from assessment of the caregiving experience, benefits and enjoyment of caregiving, personal gratification, and satisfaction, to mention a few (Cohen et al., 2002; Haley et al., 2003; Lawton, Rajagopal, Brody, & Kleban, 1992). However, no studies have linked all the independent variables mentioned with subjective wellbeing as the dependent variable, as represented in the current study.

The timeliness of this research is apposite. The vast disparity in research pertinent to the informal caregiver is apparent. Informal caregivers as well as the communities that offer them support (e.g., advocacy groups, medical institutions, social service agencies, and the general populace) seek advice, direction, and resources in handling the issues that arise for the caregiver. It was these researchers hope that the current study would contribute to the research regarding factors that can influence the wellbeing of the informal caregiver.

Purpose of the Research

The purpose of this mixed methods study was to examine the influence of self-efficacy, social support, resilience, spirituality, and leisure participation on the subjective wellbeing of informal caregivers.

Research Question

Based on the problem statement for this study, one research question was addressed: What are the significant factors that contribute to increased levels of subjective wellbeing of informal caregivers?

Hypotheses

To begin to answer the research question, the researchers developed testable statistical hypotheses. There was one null hypothesis and one alternative hypothesis for each of the predictor variables presented in this study:

$H1_0$: There is no relationship between self-efficacy and the subjective wellbeing of informal caregivers.
$H1_a$: There is a positive relationship between self-efficacy and the subjective wellbeing of informal caregivers.
$H2_0$: There is no relationship between social support and the subjective wellbeing of informal caregivers.
$H2_a$: There is a positive relationship between social support and the subjective wellbeing of informal caregivers.
$H3_0$: There is no relationship between resilience and the subjective wellbeing of informal caregivers.
$H3_a$: There is a positive relationship between resilience and the subjective wellbeing of informal caregivers.

$H4_0$: There is no relationship between spirituality and the subjective wellbeing of informal caregivers.
$H4_a$: There is a positive relationship between spirituality and the subjective wellbeing of informal caregivers.
$H5_0$: There is no relationship between leisure participation and the subjective wellbeing of informal caregivers.
$H5_a$: There is a positive relationship between leisure participation and the subjective wellbeing of informal caregivers.

DEFINITION OF TERMS

The items listed in this section may have different meanings in various contexts or other studies. To avoid confusion and misunderstanding of how these words were applied in the current research as well as to ensure the terms were understood to be specific and appropriate to the current investigation, the following definitions are provided.

Formal caregiver: "Formal caregivers including home health care providers and other professionals [who] are trained and paid for their services. Some formal caregivers are trained volunteers associated with an agency" (Family Caregiver Alliance, 2014, p. 12).

Informal caregiver: Goodhead and McDonald (2007) described an informal caregiver as those:

Caring for a friend, family member or neighbor who because of sickness, frailty or disability can't manage everyday living without help or support . . . [it] is not usually based on any formal agreement or service specifications. Informal care giving is characterized by relationships and social expectations. (p. 4)

Leisure participation: Dunn and Strain (2001) defined leisure participation as "participating in activities/interests such as regular exercise, hobbies, free time for oneself, sex life, opportunities to socialize with friends, community involvement, vacations and leisure time pursuits and activities" (p. 32).

Resilience: Gaugler, Kane, and Newcomer (2007) explained this term as "positive or successful adaptation, competence, and functioning in the face of stressful experiences" (p. 38).

Self-efficacy: Bandura (1978) defined self-efficacy as "a judgment of one's ability to execute a particular behavior pattern" (p. 240).

Social support: Findler (2000) described social support as "the extent to which a person receives assistance and help from others, and also to a sense of belonging" (p. 370). She continued to assert that there are three dimensions of social support: formal versus informal, received (objective) versus perceived (subjective), and structural versus functional. The focus in the current study was on the second dimension, concentrating on the perceived facet that highlights "the recipients' perceptions of what comes from others and their view of this support as helpful or intended as helpful" (p. 371).

Spirituality: Buck (2006) defined spirituality as "that most human of experiences that seeks to transcend self and find meaning and purpose through connection with others, nature, and/or a Supreme Being, which may or may not involve religious structures or traditions" (p. 290).

REFERENCES

Allen, S. M., & Ciambrone, D. (2003). Community care for people with disability: Blurring boundaries between formal & informal caregiver. *Qualitative Health Research*, *2*(2), 207–226. doi:10.1177/1049732302239599 PMID:12643029

Bandura, A. (1978). Reflections on self-efficacy. In S. Rachman (Ed.), *Advances in behavior research and therapy* (pp. 237–269). Oxford, UK: Pergamon.

Buck, H. G. (2006). Spirituality: Concept analysis and model development. *Holistic Nursing Practice*, *20*(6), 288–292. doi:10.1097/00004650-200611000-00006 PMID:17099417

Bulger, M. W., Wandersman, A., & Goldman, C. R. (1993). Burdens and gratifications of caregiving: Appraisal of parental care of adults with schizophrenia. *The American Journal of Orthopsychiatry*, *63*(2), 255–265. doi:10.1037/h0079437 PMID:8484431

Cohen, C. A., Colantonio, A., & Vernich, L. (2002). Positive aspects of caregiving: Rounding out the caregiver experience. *International Journal of Geriatric Psychiatry*, *17*(2), 184–188. doi:10.1002/gps.561 PMID:11813283

Dunn, N. J., & Strain, L. A. (2001). Caregivers at risk? Changes in leisure participation. *Journal of Leisure Research*, *33*(1), 32–55. doi:10.1080/00222216.2001.11949929

Findler, L. S. (2000). The role of grandparents in the social support system of mothers of children with a physical disability. *Families in Society*, *81*(4), 370–381. doi:10.1606/1044-3894.1033

Gaugler, J. E., Kane, R. L., Kane, R. A., Clay, T., & Newcomer, R. (2003). Caregiving and institutionalization of cognitively impaired older people: Utilizing dynamic predictors of change. *The Gerontologist*, *43*(2), 219–229. doi:10.1093/geront/43.2.219 PMID:12677079

Goodhead, A., & McDonald, J. (2007). *Informal caregivers literature review. A report prepared for the National Heath Committee*. Wellington, New Zealand: Health Services Centre, Victoria University of Wellington.

Haley, W. E., LaMonde, L. A., Han, B., Burton, A. M., & Schonwetter, R. (2003). Predictors of depression and life satisfaction among spousal caregivers in hospice: Application of a stress process model. *Journal of Palliative Medicine*, *6*(2), 215–224. doi:10.1089/109662103764978461 PMID:12854938

Kramer, B. J. (1997). Gain in the caregiving experience: Where are we? What next? *The Gerontologist*, *37*(2), 218–232. doi:10.1093/geront/37.2.218 PMID:9127978

Lawton, M. P., Rajagopal, D., Brody, E., & Kleban, M. H. (1992). The dynamics of caregiving for a demented elder among Black and White families. *Journal of Gerontology*, *47*(4), S156–S164. doi:10.1093/geronj/47.4.S156 PMID:1624710

Robinson, B. (1983). Validation of a caregiver strain index. *Journal of Gerontology*, *38*(3), 344–348. doi:10.1093/geronj/38.3.344 PMID:6841931

ADDITIONAL READING

Diener, Ed., Lucas, R., Schimmack, U., & Halliwell, J. (2009). *Wellbeing for public policy: Positive Psychology* (1st ed.). Oxford, UK: Oxford University Press, Inc.

Diener, Ed., & Suh, E. M. (2000). *Culture and subjective wellbeing*. Cambridge, MA: The MIT Press.

Eid, M., & Larsen, R. J. (2008). *The science of subjective wellbeing*. Guilford Publications, Inc.

Lane, R. (2001). *The loss of happiness in market democracies*. New Haven, CT: Yale University Press.

Chapter 1
Research on Subjective Wellbeing

ABSTRACT

This chapter posits that based on a careful review of extant literature, the quest to identify the factors that assist caregivers in sustaining or elevating their subjective wellbeing while providing comfort and support to care recipients is critical. In this sense, discussion in this chapter provides a rationale for the design and focus of research reported in this book, which focuses on the positive factors that elevate subjective wellbeing of informal caregivers. Thus, this chapter explores various research findings and theoretical discussion on associations between subjective wellbeing and fundamental characteristics of mental and psychical wellness of those providing care on an informal basis. These include the accentuation of self-efficacy and spirituality. It also includes the extent to which an informal caregiver receives support from others to enhance a sense of belonging to community. In addition, it further includes personal resilience of the caregiver as well as opportunities to participate in leisure activities and community involvement.

INTRODUCTION

The daily tasks of a caregiver can seem insurmountable. The quest to identify factors that assist caregivers in maintaining or elevating their subjective wellbeing while providing comfort and support to care recipients is critical. Given the criticality of these factors, this study was designed purposely to

DOI: 10.4018/978-1-5225-7452-1.ch001

examine various constructs that may aid in this pursuit. A review of literature and related research was consequently undertaken to investigate work that had been done previously in this area and to establish the rationale for the current study. However, an expansive and comprehensive review of literature and research revealed no extant studies dealing directly with the topic of the current investigation.

This chapter contains a review of the body of research and publications related to the selected topic to provide a relevant context for the focus of the current study. The researchers examined five independent variables to determine their influence on the subjective wellbeing of the informal caregiver: self-efficacy, resilience, spirituality, social support, and leisure participation. Readers should note the degrees of statistical associations between these factors and subjective wellbeing are reported in chapter three of this book.

SUBJECTIVE WELLBEING

I am determined to be cheerful and happy in whatever situation I may find myself. For I have learned that the greater part of our misery or unhappiness is determined not by our circumstances but by our disposition. Martha Washington (1789)

Since the 1800s, philosophers, scholars, and religious leaders alike have been curious about the concept of subjective wellbeing, though they had not termed the concept as such. These individuals concentrated on the emotional, mental, and physical pleasures and pains people experience. Notable philosopher, Jeremy Bentham, whose central influence was on moral philosophy and the theory of utilitarianism, also wrote on the subject of wellbeing and stated that the existence of pleasure and the lack of pain are essential components of living (Internet Encyclopedia of Philosophy, n.d.).

Empirical research into subjective wellbeing began early in the 20th century. Fluegel conducted one of the first relevant studies in 1925 on subjective wellbeing utilizing quantitative methods. He assessed the moods of nine respondents (five females and four males) by asking them to diary their emotional events. He focused on their recordings of pleasure and pain, and then quantified their reactions across moments in time. His findings reflected that individuals were more active and energetic when their moods were elevated (Fluegel, 1925, pp. 345-346). His study was further significant as it precluded modern experience sampling approaches on subjective wellbeing (Diener, Oishi, & Lucas, 2003).

Shortly after World War II, researchers began using short and simple questionnaires to ask individuals about their happiness levels and life satisfaction. These researchers wanted to reproduce representative samples of varying nationalities and chose respondents based on certain demographic criteria. The respondents were asked basic questions and were given simple response choices. Even though the questionnaires used were brief, they yielded important findings. A case in point is a 1969 study conducted by social psychologist, Norman Bradburn. The study questionnaire, albeit brief, had an influential impact across various social research disciplines. One of the more germane findings in the study was the revelation that persons with substantial family responsibilities and low income purported decreased levels of wellbeing (Bradburn, 1969).

Wilson conducted a comprehensive review on subjective wellbeing in 1967 with his research entitled, "Correlates of Avowed Happiness." He believed the theories of happiness had been stagnant since the days of the Greek philosophers. The conclusion from his 1967 study was that happy people generally possessed the following characteristics: "young, healthy, well-educated, well-paid, extroverted, optimistic, worry-free, religious, married person with high self-esteem, job morale, modest aspiration, of either sex and of a wide range of intelligence" (Wilson, 1967, p. 294). Since the time of this study and within the last several decades, structured methodical research has flourished in the field of wellbeing exploration (Oishi, Kesebir, & Diener, 2011).

The development of the term subjective wellbeing is attributed to psychologist Ed Diener, and defines how individuals perceive the quality of their lives. It comprises aspects of cognitive judgment and emotional reactions. It encompasses moods and emotions as well as assessments of a person's satisfaction with both the general and specific areas of his or her life. Diener's most noteworthy work involved his contribution to the measurement of happiness itself. He contended that an individual's happiness quotient is genetic and suggested that demographic factors only marginally affect an individual's innate happiness level. A significant portion of his research focused on three major components of subjective wellbeing: a positive affect (pleasurable feelings), a negative affect (painful feelings), and life satisfaction. Diener believed these three factors give subjective wellbeing construct validity and enable it to be measured (Diener & Diener, 1996). Waldron (2010) indicated that part of this viewpoint was based on the influx of recent studies that showed life satisfaction and happiness measures were dependable and offered a valid account people's wellbeing (Waldron, 2010).

Subjective Wellbeing and the Informal Caregiver

The world's aging population and recent advances in medicine have contributed to the surge in the need for informal caregivers (Council of State Governments, 2000). As such, explorations of issues pertaining to informal caregivers and subjective wellbeing have swelled. Since the 1970s, researchers in the fields of gerontology and medicine have produced a vast array of literature focusing on a variety of variables and the informal caregiver (George & Gwyther, 1986; Kramer, 1997; Yates, Tennstedt, & Chang, 1999; Yee & Schulz, 2000), such as employment (Stone & Short, 1990), finances (Donelan et al., 2002), and even marital concerns (Choi & Marks, 2006).

George and Gwyther (1986) conducted a study in which they examined the general wellbeing of family caregivers who were providing in-home care to memory-impaired elderly. They assessed four generic categories among this population: financial resources, mental health, physical health, and social participation. Their findings revealed in-home family caregivers reported deceased wellbeing in all the categories studied. These individuals also reported higher levels of stress and increased usage of psychotropic medications. George and Gwyther concluded this outcome was related to reduce levels of mental health and social participation. Another quantitative study performed in Australia revealed similar results. Van den Berg, Fiebig, and Hall (2014) used a relatively new analytical method that applied a fixed effect ordered logit model to analyze subjective wellbeing and found through econometric estimates that an individual who provides informal care can experience negative effects on his or her subjective wellbeing.

Burden is the term frequently used in the literature to define the negative aspects of the caregiving experience and their effect on wellbeing. The term expresses the adverse effects of caregiving on the emotional, financial, physical, psychological, and social wellbeing of the caregiver (George & Gwyther, 1986). Myriad other factors can contribute to the feeling of burden for the caregiver. One such example was provided in a study by Gaynor (1988) that showed the amount of caregiving affected the burden perceived by participants. Those who provided care for longer durations conveyed that they experienced greater burden (Gaynor, 1988). Andren and Elmståhl (2008) claimed burden to be a predictor of perceived health. Caregivers to people with dementia were asked to complete a caregiver burden scale. The final analysis showed the caregivers claiming lower burden also described better health, while those with increased burden indicated poorer health conditions.

Recently, there has been a shift in the research focus of caregiving. Not only are studies being conducted concerning the negative consequences of providing care to a caregiver's wellbeing, some researchers are examining the positive effects as well. Ashworth and Baker (2000) queried 23 caregivers between the ages 14 and 85 about their caregiving experience. The participants (40%) conveyed positive satisfaction with their care provision. In another study (McDaid, 2001), caregivers expressed that it was not the act of caring that triggered satisfaction but rather the euphoria state they felt because of providing care and doing something good.

The National Opinion Research Center (2014) conducted a survey via telephone of 1,419 Americans aged 40 or older. They primarily sought the views from this population regarding long-term care issues. The researchers discovered many individuals were caring for family members on a continuous basis. These individuals expressed that being a caregiver was a positive experience for them. They believed their role gave them the opportunity to give back to someone who had cared for them. The caregivers also expressed feeling personal growth and an amplified purpose in their own lives.

Some believed their experiences as a caregiver would be seen as a tradition of care, which could be modeled by their own children. They also reported finding benefits in their role and activities as a caregiver that contributed to a positive shift in their overall wellbeing. Haley et al. (2003) noted in their conclusions that caregivers who can identify more benefits from their role than obstacles reported lower levels of depression. The ability to perceive the caregiver experience positively can offer a sense of satisfaction and wellbeing to the caregiver even after this relationship has terminated.

Additional studies have shown that caregivers exhibited better overall wellbeing when they could identify more positive aspects of caregiving than adverse outcomes. Results of a study by Chen and Greenberg (2004) of 560 caregivers of people suffering with schizophrenia showed that since assuming their role they had discovered an inner strength. They also claimed they had developed a better insight into life and were more compassionate toward people with mental disabilities. Marsh et al. (1996) gauged the wellbeing of participants using an open-ended survey where the subjects declared their caregiver experiences caused them to reassess their lives, increased their resilience, and contributed to personal growth. Even with the expanse of new research on caregiver wellbeing and its positive correlates, comparable studies are in demand.

In summary, the impact of becoming a caregiver on subjective wellbeing can be significant (Moen, Robison, & Dempster-McClain, 1995). The negative aspects of caregiving have been exhaustively examined (Toseland, McCallion, Gerber, & Banks, 2002). As such, there is a gap in the literature addressing what factors can improve caregivers' perceptions of their lives (Pressler et al., 2013). As the caregiving phenomenon expands, mixed methods research is critical to understanding how caregivers can influence their quality of life as they embrace their role in the hopes that interventions can be developed to support this budding segment of the population (Addington-Hall & Kalra, 2001). That was the purpose of the current study.

Self-Efficacy and the Informal Caregiver

It is our duty as human beings to proceed as though the limits of our capabilities do not exist. – Pierre Teilhard de Chardin (n.d.)

Bandura (1995), the founder of the concept of *self-efficacy*, defined it as "the belief in one's capabilities to organize and execute the courses of action required to manage prospective situations" (p. 2). Simply stated, self-efficacy is a person's own belief that he or she possesses the ability to achieve his or her goals. A person's level of self-efficacy dictates how the individual feels, thinks, and motivates him or herself to successfully manage the demands of a specific situation (Zeiss, Gallagher-Thompson, Lovett, Rose, & McKibbin, 1999). Bandura explained that individuals possessing elevated levels of self-efficacy believe they have more control over their own destiny while those with decreased self-efficacy levels may often assume that they are powerless in managing their lives. Bandura (1995) emphasized that self-efficacy can be developed via four main sources of influence:

- *Mastery of experiences* is the most critical source of influence in attaining self-efficacy. The more a person succeeds at accomplishing or overcoming a challenging task, the more efficacious he or she will become, thereby increasing self-efficacy.
- *Vicarious experiences* are another significant source of influence toward reaching self-efficacy. When an individual witnesses others succeed, it empowers him or her to believe that he or she is also capable of

similar feats. This is most effective when those being observed mirror the individual.

- *Social persuasion* is yet another influential source in strengthening an individual's belief that he or she possesses the necessary skill set to succeed. If an individual is persuaded verbally that he or she can acquire the competencies to master given activities, that individual will likely exert a greater effort toward accomplishing the goal.
- *Psychological responses* have a tremendous effect on self-efficacy levels. The manner in which a person reacts to and interprets stressful situations can affect how he or she feels about his or her personal abilities in a particular situation. Bandera stated, "It is not the sheer intensity of emotional and physical reactions that is important but rather how they are perceived and interpreted." (p. 2). In other words, if an individual can alter his or her own negative emotional proclivities, he or she may be able to boost his or her self-efficacy.

As related to the role of informal caregiving, self-efficacy refers to the caregiver's belief in his or her ability to provide care for the care recipient. Several studies have been conducted to explore the significance of self-efficacy to the caregiver. Zeiss et al. (1999) purported informal caregivers who exhibit higher levels of self-efficacy claim to feel less stressed in their role. Higher self-efficacy levels allow the caregiver to better manage the disruptive behaviors sometimes exhibited by the care recipient (Rabinowitz, Mausbach, & Gallagher-Thompson, 2009).

Prior studies also showed that high self-efficacy has a direct link to experiencing the caregiver role more positively (Carbonneau, Caron, & Desrosiers, 2010). Bandura (1997) claimed that self-efficacy can be developed through mastery of experiences, vicarious experiences, social persuasion, and psychological responses. Also, establishing a connection between self-efficacy and caregiving can have realistic inferences for caregiver interventions (Carbonneau et al., 2010; Kramer, 1997).

Gilliam and Steffen (2006) alleged that caregivers with higher levels of self-efficacy view the tasks associated with their duties as missions to be mastered and not situations to be shunned. According to Bandura (1997), "A resilient sense of self-efficacy enables people to endure hardships and persevere against great odds" (p. 22) that are associated with caregiving. Bandura (2006) expounded on this theory by signifying that people with higher levels of self-efficacy are more adept at completing caregiving tasks than are those who purport lower levels of self-efficacy.

They also report reduced burnout rates, fewer maladies involving personal psychological or physical health, and enhanced wellbeing. Other studies have shown that informal caregivers with higher levels of self-efficacy claim decreases in blood pressure ratings, cardiac disease, depression levels, and perceived burden (Au et al., 2010; Gallagher, Luttik, & Jaarsma, 2011; Mausbach et al., 2012; Montoro-Rodriguez & Gallagher-Thompson, 2009; Rodríguez-Sanchez et al., 2011; Romero-Moreno et al., 2011).

It is likely that those caregivers with higher self-efficacy might be better equipped to recognize the positive aspects of the role simply because they are aware of ways to self-soothe whenever negative circumstances occur. Hellström, Nolan, and Lundh (2007) found that when caregivers and their care recipients engaged in enrichment events, this enhanced their relationship and promoted positivity around the caregiving experience. Bandura (1997) asserted that caregivers with increased levels of self-efficacy exhibit more motivation to act on their surroundings in a manner that promotes positive wellbeing. These individuals may seek out mutually enjoyable events that can be shared between themselves and the care recipient. This can enrich the relationship between them while also fostering an improved sense of efficiency and contentment in the caregiving role.

Caregiver self-efficacy is a multi-layered variable that vacillates over time according to the caregiver's particular situation (Bandura, 1977). A strong sense of self-efficacy can make the experience of caregiving less stressful (Bandura, 1981). The skillful use of coping strategies can help to improve the self-efficacy of the caregiver and enhance his or her quality of life (Welch & West, 1995). It is critical to continue the examination of the effect of this variable on the caregiving experience for the continued development of effective intervention programs.

Spirituality and the Informal Caregiver

We are not human beings having a spiritual experience; we are spiritual beings having a human experience. – Pierre Teilhard de Chardin (n.d.)

Buck (2006) explained *spirituality* as "that most human of experiences that seeks to transcend self and find meaning and purpose through connection with others, nature, and/or a Supreme Being, which may or may not involve religious structures or traditions" (p. 289). The informal caregiver can find solace through his or her spiritual beliefs as he or she experiences the caregiver journey. Results of a 1999 qualitative study conducted with African American caregivers at Boston University revealed that the participants claimed they were primarily sustained by faith and inner strength (Poindexter, Linsk, & Warner, 1999). They asserted that their most vital support system was not other people, but God. They explained that their spiritual beliefs were their major source of sustenance and contended that these values were critical in helping them cope with their current challenging situation (Poindexter et al., 1999).

Some researchers describe this coping mechanism as the *faith factor* (Matthews & Clark, 1999). The faith factor has been reviewed from various angles, ranging from behavioral (service attendance, frequency of prayer) and descriptive (denominational preference) to more personalized aspects such as the intensity of one's beliefs, self-report of a person's religiosity, the significance of religion to an individual's life, the reassurances a person experiences via religion, and religious dedication and orthodoxy. Even though findings have varied somewhat from study to study, in general it appears there is a positive association between religion and mental and physical wellbeing (Chang, Noonan, & Tennstedt, 1998). The findings can be positively viewed, particularly by the spiritually-centered caregiver.

A strong spiritual center can be significant for some individuals when confronted with highly stressful situations (Taylor, 2006; Tuck, 2004). The last section of this chapter will tackle the positive impact of spirituality on subjective wellbeing from a cognitive development perspective. In one study, those who professed allegiance to God claimed that their spiritual belief provided a source of strength in handling the challenges related to caregiving (Borrayo, Goldwaser, Vacha-Haase, & Hepburn, 2007). This seemed particularly prominent among minority caregivers when considering the views they often expressed regarding their caregiving experience. For example, a quantitative study conducted by Hodge and Sun (2012) into the role of spirituality as a predictor of positive aspects of caregiving revealed positive correlations. A total of 209 Latino caregivers of family members with Alzheimer's were recruited from multiple community organizations in cities within California, Florida, and Pennsylvania. The researchers measured spirituality using three indicators: prayer/meditation, religious service attendance, and spiritual coping.

They also used the Positive Aspects of Caregiving (PAC) nine-item scale to assess perceptions of benefits within the caregiving context. They discovered spirituality to be positively associated with PAC scores. Similar results were noted by Nápoles, Chadiha, Eversley, and John (2010), who examined the ethnic differences in dementia caregivers' experiences. The cultural differences most frequently documented among the African American population compared to the groups of Latinos, Chinese, and European Americans were "better psychosocial health, more positive appraisals of caregiving, and greater spirituality or use of prayer" (p. 5). This suggests spirituality plays a prominent role in overall wellbeing among minority populations.

Guberman, Maheu, and Maillé (1992) asserted that the religious beliefs of family caregivers were closely linked to the incentive to care for infirmed and intellectually challenged family members. Faver (2004) discovered a similar finding between family caregivers and their religious beliefs. They professed their motivation to care for family members stemmed from their strong spiritual principles. Many informal caregivers contend that their spiritual connection affects all their decisions and actions as a caregiver. This claim was supported by a study conducted by Montgomery (1991), who termed this feeling as the *spiritual transcendence* characteristics expressed by many caregivers.

Numerous studies have shown that a caregiver's spiritual beliefs can be the cornerstone of his or her conviction and strength when dealing with the challenges associated with caregiving responsibilities (Brotherson & Soderquist, 2002). Some caregivers allege that their spiritual connectedness provides them greater resolve to handle the daily trials of their role (Pargament, 2010). Overall, the research illustrates that such convictions can be positively more significant among certain cultures, thereby helping them cope with the stressors of providing care to someone who is infirmed (Dilworth-Anderson, Williams, & Gibson, 2002).

Social Support and the Informal Caregiver

No one is useless in this world who lightens the burden of others. (Dickens, 1865)

Findler (2000) described *social support* as "the extent to which a person receives assistance and help from others, and also to a sense of belonging" (p. 370). Findler (2000) explained that there are three dimensions of social support: formal versus informal, received (objective) versus perceived (subjective), and structural versus functional. These dimensions have some commonalities while still offering vastly unique aid to the care provider. Scholars believe the resources from social support aid in reducing a host of negative outcomes for caregivers (Williams et al., 2008). The support received from informal networks can alleviate the negative aspects of caregiving such as emotional distress, health concerns, and economic strain (Miller et al., 2001). Structural support can be represented via instrumental aid (e.g., financial help) or spiritual guidance (Findler, 2000). Formal support systems might provide help via home health care professionals, long-term care options, mental health assistance, and monetary support, to mention a few (Williams & Dilworth-Anderson, 2002). While the type of social support deemed most effective is in dispute (Miller et al., 2001), researchers agree that having access to different forms of social support is beneficial (Brand, Barry, & Gallagher, 2014).

Over the past few decades, most studies conducted revealed evidence of a substantial relationship between social support and a caregiver's wellbeing (Atienza, Collins, & King, 2001; Chang, Brecht, & Carter, 2001; Dilworth-Anderson et al., 2002; Franks & Stephens, 1996; Gerdner, Hall, & Buckwalter, 1996). Redinbaugh, MacCallum, and Kiecolt-Glaser conducted one such study in 1995. In their 3-year longitudinal study they evaluated 103 family caregivers yearly for depression and discovered that those caregivers complaining of elevated levels of depression also claimed an increased number of traumatic life events coupled with decreased levels of positive social support.

In an earlier study, Kiecolt-Glaser, Dura, Speicher, Trask, and Glaser (1991) discovered that spousal caregivers claiming they had little to no social support had the largest number of negative changes to their immune systems at follow-up medical visits. Results of a study conducted in 1996 by Franks and Stephens revealed that the caregivers who had better emotional and social support generally reported decreased levels of depression and increased life satisfaction. In 1998, Rapp, Shumaker, Schmidt, Naughton, and Anderson discovered that a caregiver's social resourcefulness was correlated with wellbeing.

These types of studies continued to flourish during the next decade with research performed by Lévesque, Ducharme, and Lachance (2000). Their 1-year longitudinal study of informal caregivers of institutionalized patients showed that those caregivers who received more formal support had a lower propensity of reports involving psychological distress. Similarly, Bauer et al. (2000) established that the stressors experienced by caregivers decreased over time among those who sought and received social support. Likewise, Gupta and Pillai (2000) found that as a caregiver's social network expanded, his or her burden levels decreased significantly.

The support received can be from associates, business colleagues, family members, friends, or neighbors. Most important is that the caregiver believes he or she is able to access his or her social network for assistance whenever necessary (Schwarzer, Dunkel-Schetter, & Kemeny, 1994; Shenk, 2014).

Another example of this assertion can be found in the study conducted by Kaufman, Kosberg, Leeper, and Tang (2010) of 141 African American and White dementia caregivers living in rural Alabama. The participants, as a whole, claimed that the high level of social support they received from neighbors, family, and friends helped alleviate the burden associated with providing care for an infirmed family member. Similarly, additional health benefits have been reported by those caregivers who receive ample social support (Thorsteinsson & James, 1999; Uno, Uchino, & Smith, 2002). Generally, the research shows that social support (either received or perceived) is essential to helping caregivers manage the life stressors they often encounter (Lakey & Cronin, 2008; Uchino, 2009).

Several studies have shown social support to be a meaningful influence on the wellbeing levels of informal caregivers (Gupta & Pillai, 2000; Haley et al., 1996; Majerovitz, 2007; Pillemer & Suitor, 2000). Whether the support is actually received or perceived seems not to diminish the significance of its effect on a caregiver's wellbeing (Thompson, Futterman, Gallagher-Thompson, Rose, & Lovett, 1993). Research highlights that social support has substantial health benefits to a caregiver's psychological and psychological wellbeing (Gupta & Pillai, 2000; Thorsteinsson & James, 1999; Uno et al., 2002). This influence appears to be equally significant in both urban and rural settings among caregivers (Kaufman et al., 2010).

Resilience and the Informal Caregiver

Life doesn't get easier or more forgiving; we get stronger and more resilient. (Maraboli, 2009)

Gaugler et al. (2007) defined the term *resilience* as "positive or successful adaption, competence, and functioning in the face of stressful experience" (p. 38). Their exploration into how resilience affects caregivers showed that a majority of the prior studies conducted often focused on the "wear and tear hypothesis" (Gaugler et al., 2007, p. 38), which emphasized how at-home care provided by an informal caregiver is associated with a plethora of negative consequences. However, newer studies began to be conducted to explore how caregivers were positively adapting to their circumstances. The findings seem to support that the presence of resilience helps caregivers remain stable or decreases the mental strain often linked to the caregiving experience (Donnellan, Bennett, & Soulsby, 2015, 2016; Gaugler, Davey, Pearlin, & Zarit, 2000; Wilks & Croom, 2008).

The individual who withstands obstacles and continues to persevere is considered resilient (Garity, 1997; Greene et al., 2002; Werner & Smith, 2001). A plethora of research has been conducted on the concept of resilience and its effects on children. Yet, in the field of gerontology, this theory is still in its infancy, but has important implications.

Garity (1997) conducted one of the earlier studies pertaining to caregivers and resilience. She evaluated 76 participants from an Alzheimer's Association support group in Eastern Massachusetts. She sought to study the relationships among learning style, resilience factors, stress level, and the manner in which these caregivers coped. The purpose of Garity's query was to offer more specific educational interventions for support groups of caregivers. She also wanted to identify distinct characteristics associated with a more resilient caregiver. Garity believed this information to be very useful but acknowledged that the cross-sectional study design she used limited the generalizability of her findings because the relationship indicated in the findings could not generalize to caregivers outside the study parameters. Nevertheless, Garity (1997) discovered that individuals with higher levels of self-reliance, independence, determination, mastery, adaptability, and balance used coping strategies to draw on the positive aspects of caregiving and refused to be overwhelmed by their circumstances. This study denotes the significance of individual characteristics associated with resilience. Resilience was also positively correlated with other coping mechanisms such as distancing and organized problem-solving. Garity (1997) believed the ability to identify these features in a person would be useful in predicting caregiver outcomes.

Ross, Holliman, and Dixon (2003) conducted a qualitative exploratory study of Alzheimer's caregivers to identify common themes, activities, and characteristics associated with resilient caregivers. The sample consisted of 23 participants caring for Alzheimer's patients. These caregivers were asked questions using the Caregiver Resilience Instrument, which consists of four items. Caregivers who were deemed more resilient revealed the following factors as most influential: access to a good support system, appreciating the number of years as a caregiver, being physically active with hobbies, finding humor in a situation, staying spiritually connected, and maintaining one's own identity. These findings support that there are correlations among caregivers' personal characteristics, their coping behavior, and resilience.

A caregiver's level of resilience can be the deciding factor in whether he or she remains as a caregiver or opts for institutionalization. Gaugler, Kane, Kane, Clay, and Newcomer (2003) conducted a study of informal caregivers of persons with dementia and discovered that their findings were consistent with those of earlier studies. For example, results reflected that perceived burden, self-rated health, and community-based service usage were significant predictors of early nursing home placement. Additionally, shifts in both the care recipient and caregivers' instrumental activities of daily living might cause expedited institutionalization. These findings accentuate the need to integrate care recipient and caregiver invention programs to meet the needs of each party.

A better understanding of resilience as it pertains to the informal caregiver will greatly serve society as it continues to encounter the upsurge in the need for this populace. The development of educational or intervention programs to elevate caregivers' resilience levels will be significant as they encounter the adversity often associated with their role (Payne & Morbey, 2013). Early research reflected that resilient caregivers exhibit high levels of self-reliance, independence, and determination, and consistently draw on the positive aspects of caregiving by refusing to be overwhelmed by their circumstances, and therefore fare better (Garity, 1997). These personal characteristics, a solid support system, remaining physically active, staying spiritually connected, and maintaining comical sensibilities will be invaluable to persons having to assume the caregiver position (Ross et al., 2003). This knowledge will also be important to the communities of people and caregiver organizations that assist this populace, as it can provide each party with the skills and resources needed to navigate this evolving terrain.

Leisure Participation and the Informal Caregiver

If you are losing your leisure, Look out! You are losing your soul. (Pearsall Smith (n.d.)

Dunn and Strain (2001) defined *leisure participation* as "participating in activities/interests such as regular exercise, hobbies, free time for oneself, sex life, opportunities to socialize with friends, community involvement, vacations and leisure time pursuits and activities" (p. 32).

The responsibilities of informal caregivers can often be the precipice for chaos to their leisure lifestyle. Their leisure pursuits are often derailed and sometimes extinguished entirely because of the demands of the occupation. Results of a study conducted by White-Means and Chang (1994) showed that variances in the caregiver's sociodemographic characteristics, economic variables, and caregiver settings significantly affect the caregiver's leisure. Additionally, the day-to-day duties that the caregiver performs can cause him or her to have less time for leisure activities. As a result, the overwrought caregiver can experience emotional and physical stress and less satisfaction with life overall.

Oftentimes, caregivers find themselves *sandwiched* between tending to the needs of an ailing parent and caring for a child under the age of 18. They may also be employed either full- or part-time. The standard profile of an informal caregiver is a person who is 49 years of age and spends approximately 24.4 hours weekly providing care to the care recipient, and the daily routine allows limited time for leisure pursuits (Family Caregiver Alliance, 2016). The usual time sanctioned for leisure participation is frequently deleted from the weekly agenda once someone assumes an informal caregiver role. Ironically, devoting time to leisure activities can offer the most benefit to the informal caregiver by promoting positive feelings, providing external stimulation, and encouraging socialization (Baker, Cahalin, Gerst, & Burr, 2005).

Caregivers often express feeling most challenged by the havoc and the demands of caregiving duties on their free time. King et al. (2005) conducted a study of approximately 3,000 middle-aged women and found that caregiving responsibilities and lack of energy ranked in the top percentile (2 of 4) of barriers to these individuals being physically active. To expound on the White-Means and Chang (1994) research, the results also showed a 62% probability that caregiving responsibilities will restrict a family's leisure time. King et al. (2005) further contended that the obligations had an 81% probability of compromising personal free time, practically voiding the caregiver of any leisure enjoyment. This loss of leisure time holds significant concern for many caregivers. Scharlach (1994) investigated the aspects of caregiving that were most challenging to the caregivers and found that lack of personal time ranked second of the seven issues most pertinent to caregivers. The National Family Caregivers Association performed another study in 1998 that showed caregivers chose the loss of leisure second out of 10 aspects as the facet of their caregiving experience to which they had the most difficulty adjusting.

Moreover, there is significant research that supports the position that a loss of leisure activities is closely related to depressive symptoms, elevated stress levels, and the development or aggravation of other health issues (Wakui, Saito, Agree, & Kai, 2012). Staight and Harvey (1990) revealed an increase in depression scores when caregivers attested to shortened sessions for relaxation. Additional studies have also revealed limited activity to be a contributor to depression (Nieboer et al., 1998; Williamson, Shaffer, & Schulz, 1998) within the informal caregiver community. Silliman (1993) discovered a connection among the levels of restriction in social activities for caregivers and their views of their own wellbeing. Additional empirical evidence has generally indicated that low levels of pleasant and social activities are associated with poorer caregiver wellbeing (Cook, Pearson, & Ahrens, 1997; Gallagher-Thompson et al., 2000; Kramer & Thompson, 2002; Rivera, Rose, Futterman, Lovett, & Gallagher-Thompson, 1991; Thompson et al., 1993). Cannuscio et al. (2004), in a cross-sectional study of over 61,000 female caregivers, found that the more hours in a week these caregivers spent performing their responsibilities, the more they were prone to exhibit increased symptoms of depression. Some researchers claimed that a reduction in leisure activity can be linked to emotional stress, depression, and reduced life satisfaction among caregivers (Losada et al., 2010; Mausbach, Patterson, & Grant, 2008; White-Means & Chang, 1994).

Caregivers often comment that leisure or personal time can be abandoned because their responsibilities to the care recipient outweigh their own enjoyment (Hughes & Keller, 1992; Sisk, 2000). However, the research shows otherwise. Iso-Ahola (1994) posited that participating in leisure contributes to improved mental and physical health. His research emphasized that leisure has a positive effect on several aspects of life, including temperament, wellbeing, self-esteem, and reducing loneliness. Additionally, in an earlier study by Coleman and Iso-Ahola (1993), leisure was attributed to easing stressful life experiences, which can improve the ability to cope.

Wakui et al. (2012) used a multivariate regression analysis of data from 727 family caregivers of elderly Japanese citizens and found interesting results. The researchers explored whether the frequency and type of activity were more significant to improved psychological wellbeing among family caregivers. It appeared that engagement in home activities (as opposed to outside leisure pursuits) garnered lower scores on burden and depression and reflected greater care satisfaction tallies. Schryer, Mock, Hilbrecht, Lero, and Smale (2016) conducted a study to examine how the use of leisure facilities (e.g., cultural centers, parks, sporting arenas, libraries, etc.) might affect the mental and physical wellbeing of caregivers. The results revealed that more frequent visits to these types of facilities improved both the mental and physical wellbeing of these caregivers. This suggests that continued access to leisure infrastructure is critical in supporting wellbeing among caregivers. Schüz et al. (2015) purported that many informal caregivers offer assistance to dementia patients. They claimed that the caregiver population is often at a higher risk for mental health problems than others. They examined whether perceived change in leisure activities could cause a reduction in stress and mental health issues for dementia caregivers. They hypothesized that group-based leisure activities might guard against these negative effects. A participant pool of 346 dementia caregivers between the ages of 18 and 82 participated in the study. The data were analyzed using multiple regression statistics and results showed that apparent changes in leisure activities, particularly engaging in activities that included self-help group interactions or participation in social activities, mitigated the negative effects of caregiving.

Even though research illustrates that a lack of leisure activities can be more detrimental to the caregiver's physical and psychological wellbeing, caregivers often express that they believe taking time for leisure enjoyment is not significant (King et al., 2005; Scharlach, 1994; Sisk, 2000; White-Means & Chang, 1994). There is substantial research that debates this stance, emphasizing that leisure pursuits can improve a caregiver's overall wellbeing (Roberts, Halpin-Healy, McGinnis, & Noble, 2014; Schüz et al., 2015; Wakui et al., 2012). The support of this position has been repeatedly examined and seems to emphasize that when caregivers remain leisurely active and connected to their communities, they can abate a variety of illnesses (Iso-Ahola, 1994).

A MORAL DEVELOPMENT PERSPECTIVE

Our assessment of the contributions of Lawrence Kohlberg's theory of moral development to an understanding of spiritually-beliefs inspired right actions that enhance subjective wellbeing proceeds from Buck (2006)'s definitions of spirituality. Buck (2006) offers an account of spirituality that focuses on the transcending feature of human spirituality that shifts the emphasis away from the accentuation of individual self needs to finding meaning and purpose in connection with others, nature or a Supreme Being. This perspective tends to align with Kohlberg's post-conventional stage of moral reasoning (*Stage 6: The universal ethical-principle orientation*). Thus, the universal ethical principle orientation offers a conception of justice that allows us to treat the claims of all parties in an impartial manner, respecting the basic dignity, of all people as individuals. The principles of justice enshrined in this orientation presuppose universality of the type that confirms to the Golden Rule and Kant's categorical imperative (Langford, 1995). Indeed, Kant's metaphysics allows us through the operation of the universalizability principle to use reason to give content to morality (Appiah, 2003). In fact, in the *Groundwork of the Metaphysic of Morals* Kant argued that this was the only categorical imperative from which all moral principles derived (p.197).

Contrary to Kohlberg's early stages, such as stage 2 (*the instrumental relativist orientation*) in which right action consists of what instrumentally satisfies one's own needs, right action in the post-conventional stage (6) is defined by a decision of conscience in accordance with self-chosen ethical principles. In the world of practice, and in the actual Heinz dilemma, people can assume a Rawlsian type "veil of ignorance" acting as if they do not know which role they will eventually occupy (Kolhberg, 1971). Thus, the emphasis for Kohlberg is not whether one answers "yes" or "no", to the dilemma, but to understand the reasoning behind one's answer (Kolhberg, 1971). Kolhberg's (1963, p.19) interview consists of a series of dilemmas, one of which is rewritten here as follows:

Heinz Steals the Drug

In Europe, a woman was near death from a special kind of cancer. There was one drug the doctors thought might save her. It was a radium that a druggist in the same town had recently discovered. The drug was expensive to make, but the druggist was charging ten times what the drug cost him to make. He paid $200 for the radium and charged $2,000 for a small dose of what the drug cost him to make. The sick woman's husband, Heinz, went to everyone he knew to borrow the money, but he could only get together about $1,000 which is half of what it cost. He told the druggist that his wife was dying and asked him to sell it cheaper or let him pay later. But the druggist said: "No, I discovered the drug and "I'm going to make money from it." So Heinz got desperate and broke into the man's store to steal the drug for his wife. Should the husband have done that?

These researchers note that the ethical dilemma itself reflects much deeply our essential research objective, which aims to explicate the variables that affect subjective wellbeing of a sample of (n=36) informal caregivers through the desire to make manifest an ethic of care. Based on a critical review of Kohlberg's account of moral theory, these researchers observed that an underlying assumption of his theory is the assumption that humans are inherently communicative, capable of reason and possess a desire to understand others and the world around them (Kohlberg, 1981; William, 1985).

Like the formal nature of Kant's categorical imperative, Kohlberg also adopts an account of formalism in which the form and structure of moral arguments are independent of the content of those arguments. Moral reasoning is regarded as reasoning about first order norms that sit above moral edits or moral rules (Langford, 1995). Kohlberg's approach was later interpreted by Rest (Epitropaki, Butcher & Milner, 2002, p.305) as a sequential process ranging from more simpler to more complex cognitive structures focusing on greater degrees of voluntary cooperation implicit in each stage.

Readers should note, however, that developmental changes are not so much about speeding up progression from lower to upper stages, but more about avoiding cognitive retardation. Thus, the concept of *decalage* has been put forward by Kohlberg and Mayer (Power, Higgins & Kohlberg, 1989). This concept focuses more on the depth and breadth of development rather than on its rate of progression between developmental stages. Its unit of analysis is the whole person including cognitive and affective dimensions (p.18). Burnyeat (cited in Nucci, 1989) supports this strand in Kohlberg's overarching theoretical scheme and the three levels of ethical development he argues exists in Aristotle's *Nicomachean Ethics*. Each of these levels are said to have distinctive cognitive and motivational characteristics. They respond to the soul, the appetites, spirit and reasons (p.133). Aristotle's levels are said, it is argued, to bear a striking resemblance to pre-conventional, conventional and post-conventional levels in Kohlberg's theory of moral development.

There are several criticisms in the psychology of human development literature that contest the "Ethnocentrism" of Kohlberg's theory (Heibrum & Georges, 1990, p.595). Also, Carol Gilligan (1993) raises strong objections to the universality of Kohlberg's conception of maturity as embodied in post-conventional morality. Gilligan (p.19) notes that "when one begins with the study of women and derives developmental constructs from their lives, the outline of moral conception different from Freud, Piaget, or Kohlberg begins to emerge and informs a different conception of development." Galligan developed an alternative theory of moral development that does not focus on the value of justice, but rather on the ethics of caring.

Based on these suppositions, an alternative hypothesis could be considered that views the value or ethic of caring for one's love ones, when they are most in need, as a spiritual manifestation of justice anchored on commitments to universal ethical principles under the rubric of post-conventional morality. In this sense, these researchers argue that the correct and fair solution to the Heinz dilemma posited above, which argues that a sick wife must be saved, requires not only impartiality but the principle that everyone is given full and equal respect, especially family members going through moments of crisis in their lives. Such support may include care and assistance rendered to those in need by family members occupying the roles of informal caregivers.

These researchers propose that executing moral action on this basis presupposes an action that lies in conformity with one's spiritual and religious duty. The researchers further propose that perhaps this conclusion offers an illumination as to why-----caregivers tend to perceive a strong and positive connection between religious or spiritual orientation----as one of the best means of exercising agency, and thereby improving subjective wellbeing of the subject.

CONCLUSION

In summary, the literature review focused on studies that examined the subjective wellbeing of informal caregivers and the five factors of self-efficacy, social support, spirituality, leisure participation, and resilience. These studies revealed the need to further explore the caregiver phenomenon. There is consensus that the role of caregiving can be daunting. Caregivers often become so absorbed with the duties of providing care that they often neglect to maintain their own wellbeing. The responsibility of caring for an infirmed individual can cause disruption to a caregiver's physiological and psychological wellbeing that can last for weeks, months, or even years. This can be detrimental to the caregiver, his or her family, and the care recipient. Therefore, it is imperative to identify factors that may positively influence the subjective wellbeing of informal caregivers. It is also imperative to contextualize these factors in terms of a broad range of social and moral theories that provide understanding about how to integrate cognitive and affective variables in our essential models of analyses.

REFERENCES

Addington-Hall, J., & Kalra, L. (2001). Who should measure quality of life? *British Medical Journal*, *322*(7299), 1417–1420. doi:10.1136/bmj.322.7299.1417 PMID:11397754

Andren, S., & Elmståhl, S. (2008). The relationship between caregiver burden, caregivers' perceived health and their sense of coherence in caring for elders with dementia. *Journal of Clinical Nursing*, *17*(6), 790–799. doi:10.1111/j.1365-2702.2007.02066.x PMID:18279282

Appiah, A. A. (2003). *Thinking it through: An introduction to contemporary philosophy*. Oxford, UK: Oxford University Press.

Ashworth, M., & Baker, A. H. (2000). 'Time and space': Carers' views about respite care. *Health & Social Care in the Community*, *8*(1), 50–56. doi:10.1046/j.1365-2524.2000.00221.x PMID:11560674

Atienza, A. A., Collins, R., & King, A. C. (2001). The mediating effects of situational control on social support and mood following a stressor: A prospective study of dementia caregivers in their natural environments. *The Journals of Gerontology. Series B, Psychological Sciences and Social Sciences*, *56*(3), S129–S139. doi:10.1093/geronb/56.3.S129 PMID:11316838

Au, A., Lau, K.-M., Sit, E., Cheung, G., Lai, M.-K., Wong, S. K. A., & Fok, D. (2010). The role of self-efficacy in the Alzheimer's family caregiver stress process: A partial mediator between physical health and depressive symptoms. *Clinical Gerontologist*, *33*(4), 298–315. doi:10.1080/07317115.2010.502817

Baker, L. A., Cahalin, L. P., Gerst, K., & Burr, J. A. (2005). Productive activities and subjective wellbeing among older adults: The influence of number of activities and time commitment. *Social Indicators Research*, *73*(3), 431–458. doi:10.100711205-005-0805-6

Bandura, A. (1977). Self-efficacy: Toward a unifying theory of behavioral change. *Psychological Review*, *84*(2), 191–215. doi:10.1037/0033-295X.84.2.191 PMID:847061

Bandura, A. (1995). Exercise of personal and collective efficacy in changing societies. *Self-Efficacy in Changing Societies*, *15*, 334.

Bandura, A. (1997). *Self-efficacy: The exercise of control*. New York, NY: W.H. Freeman and Company.

Bandura, A. (2006). Guide for constructing self-efficacy scales. In F. Pajares & T. Urdan (Eds.), *Self-efficacy beliefs of adolescents* (pp. 308–337). Charlotte, NC: Information Age Publishing.

Bauer, M. E., Vedhara, K., Perks, P., Wilcock, G. K., Lightman, S. L., & Shanks, N. (2000). Chronic stress in caregivers of dementia patients is associated with reduced lymphocyte sensitivity to glucocorticoids. *Journal of Neuroimmunology*, *103*(1), 84–92. doi:10.1016/S0165-5728(99)00228-3 PMID:10674993

Borrayo, E. A., Goldwaser, G., Vacha-Haase, T., & Hepburn, K. W. (2007). An inquiry into Latino caregivers' experience caring for older adults with Alzheimer's disease and related dementias. *Journal of Applied Gerontology*, *26*(5), 486–505. doi:10.1177/0733464807305551

Bradburn, N. M. (1969). *The structure of psychological wellbeing*. Chicago, IL: Aldine.

Brand, C., Barry, L., & Gallagher, S. (2014). Social support mediates the association between benefit finding and quality of life in caregivers. *Journal of Health Psychology*. doi:10.1177/1359105314547244 PMID:25205775

Brotherson, S. E., & Soderquist, J. (2002). Coping with a child's death: Spiritual issues and therapeutic implications. *Journal of Family Psychotherapy*, *13*(1-2), 53–86. doi:10.1300/J085v13n01_04

Buck, H. G. (2006). Spirituality: Concept analysis and model development. *Holistic Nursing Practice*, *20*(6), 288–292. doi:10.1097/00004650-200611000-00006 PMID:17099417

Cannuscio, C. C., Colditz, G. A., Rimm, E. B., Berkman, L. F., Jones, C. P., & Kawachi, I. (2004). Employment status, social ties, and caregivers' mental health. *Social Science & Medicine*, *58*(7), 1247–1256. doi:10.1016/S0277-9536(03)00317-4 PMID:14759673

Carbonneau, H., Caron, C., & Desrosiers, J. (2010). Development of a conceptual framework of positive aspects of caregiving in dementia. *Dementia (London)*, *9*(3), 327–353. doi:10.1177/1471301210375316

Chang, B. H., Noonan, A. E., & Tennstedt, S. L. (1998). The role of religion/spirituality in coping with caregiving for disabled elders. *The Gerontologist*, *38*(4), 463–470. doi:10.1093/geront/38.4.463 PMID:9726133

Chen, F. P., & Greenberg, J. S. (2004). A positive aspect of caregiving: The influence of social support on caregiving gains for family members of relatives with schizophrenia. *Community Mental Health Journal*, *40*(5), 423–435. doi:10.1023/B:COMH.0000040656.89143.82 PMID:15529476

Choi, H., & Marks, N. F. (2006). Transition to caregiving, marital disagreement, and psychological wellbeing: A prospective US national study. *Journal of Family Issues*, *27*(12), 1701–1722. doi:10.1177/0192513X06291523

Coleman, D., & Iso-Ahola, S. E. (1993). Leisure and health: The role of social support and self-determination. *Journal of Leisure Research, 25*(2), 111–128. doi:10.1080/00222216.1993.11969913

Cook, J. M., Pearson, J. L., & Ahrens, A. H. (1997). General and specific events and depressive symptoms in Alzheimer's disease caregivers. *American Journal of Alzheimer's Disease and Other Dementias, 12*(1), 32–34. doi:10.1177/153331759701200107

Council of State Governments. (2000). *Signs of the times – Midwest demographic trends and their implications for public policy*. Retrieved from http://www.csg.org/knowledgecenter/docs/mw-Signs.pdf

Crain, W. C. (1985). *Theories of development*. Prentice-Hall. Available at: http://faculty.plts.gpnce/html/kpjberg.htm

Dickens, C. (1865). *Doctor marigold*. Fredonia, NY: Fredonia Books.

Dilworth-Anderson, P., Williams, I. C., & Gibson, B. E. (2002). Issues of race, ethnicity, and culture in caregiving research: A 20-year review (1980–2000). *The Gerontologist, 42*(2), 237–272. doi:10.1093/geront/42.2.237 PMID:11914467

Donelan, K., Hill, C. A., Hoffman, C., Scoles, K., Feldman, P. H., Levine, C., & Gould, D. (2002). Challenged to care: Informal caregivers in a changing health system. *Health Affairs, 21*(4), 222–231. doi:10.1377/hlthaff.21.4.222 PMID:12117133

Donnellan, W. J., Bennett, K. M., & Soulsby, L. K. (2015). What are the factors that facilitate or hinder resilience in older spousal dementia carers? A qualitative study. *Aging & Mental Health, 19*(10), 932–939. doi:10.1080/13607863.2014.977771 PMID:25410637

Dunn, N. J., & Strain, L. A. (2001). Caregivers at risk? Changes in leisure participation. *Journal of Leisure Research, 33*(1), 32–55. doi:10.1080/00222216.2001.11949929

Epitropaki, O., Butcher, Y., & Miller, C. (2002). Transformational leadership and moral reasoning. *The Journal of Applied Psychology, 87*(2), 304–311. doi:10.1037/0021-9010.87.2.304 PMID:12002958

Family Caregiver Alliance. (2016). *Caregiver statistics: Demographics*. Retrieved from https://www.caregiver.org/caregiver-statistics-demographics

Faver, C. A. (2004). Relational spirituality and social caregiving. *Social Work*, *49*(2), 241–249. doi:10.1093w/49.2.241 PMID:15124964

Findler, L. S. (2000). The role of grandparents in the social support system of mothers of children with a physical disability. *Families in Society*, *81*(4), 370–381. doi:10.1606/1044-3894.1033

Galligan, C. (1993). *In a different voice: Psychological theory and women's development*. Cambridge, MA: Harvard University Press.

Garity, J. (1997). Stress, learning style, resilience factors, and ways of coping in Alzheimer family caregivers. *American Journal of Alzheimer's Disease and Other Dementias*, *12*(4), 171–178. doi:10.1177/153331759701200405

Gaugler, J. E., Kane, R. L., Kane, R. A., Clay, T., & Newcomer, R. (2003). Caregiving and institutionalization of cognitively impaired older people: Utilizing dynamic predictors of change. *The Gerontologist*, *43*(2), 219–229. doi:10.1093/geront/43.2.219 PMID:12677079

Gaugler, J. E., Kane, R. L., & Newcomer, R. (2007). Resilience and transitions from dementia caregiving. *The Journals of Gerontology. Series B, Psychological Sciences and Social Sciences*, *62*(1), 38–P44. doi:10.1093/geronb/62.1.P38 PMID:17284556

Guberman, N., Maheu, P., & Maillé, C. (1992). Women as family caregivers: Why do they care? *The Gerontologist*, *32*(5), 607–617. doi:10.1093/geront/32.5.607 PMID:1427272

Gupta, R., & Pillai, V. K. (2000). Caregiver burden in South Asian families: A systems theory perspective. *Journal of Ethnic & Cultural Diversity in Social Work*, *9*(1-2), 41–53. doi:10.1300/J051v09n01_03

Haley, W. E., LaMonde, L. A., Han, B., Burton, A. M., & Schonwetter, R. (2003). Predictors of depression and life satisfaction among spousal caregivers in hospice: Application of a stress process model. *Journal of Palliative Medicine*, *6*(2), 215–224. doi:10.1089/109662103764978461 PMID:12854938

Heibrun, A. B., & Georges, M. (1990). The measurement of principled morality by the Kohlberg moral dilemma questionnaire. *Journal of Personality Assessment*, *5*(1&2), 183–194. doi:10.1080/00223891.1990.9674057 PMID:2231238

Hellström, I., Nolan, M., & Lundh, U. (2007). Sustaining couplehood: Spouses' strategies for living positively with dementia. *Dementia (London)*, *6*(3), 383–409. doi:10.1177/1471301207081571

Hodge, D. R. (2003). The Intrinsic Spirituality Scale: A new six-item instrument for assessing the salience of spirituality as a motivational construct. *Journal of Social Service Research*, *30*(1), 41–61. doi:10.1300/J079v30n01_03

Hodge, D. R., & Sun, F. (2012). Positive feelings of caregiving among Latino Alzheimer's family caregivers: Understanding the role of spirituality. *Aging & Mental Health*, *16*(6), 689–698. doi:10.1080/13607863.2012.678481 PMID:22512416

Hughes, S., & Keller, M. J. (1992). Leisure education – A coping strategy for family caregivers. *Journal of Gerontological Social Work*, *19*(1), 115–128. doi:10.1300/J083v19n01_07

Internet Encyclopedia of Philosophy. (n.d.). *Jeremy Bentham (1748—1832)*. Retrieved from http://www.iep.utm.edu/bentham/

Iso-Ahola, S. E. (1994). Leisure lifestyle and health. *Leisure and Mental Health*, *1*, 42–60.

Kaufman, A. V., Kosberg, J. I., Leeper, J. D., & Tang, M. (2010). Social support, caregiver burden, and life satisfaction in a sample of rural African American and White caregivers of older persons with dementia. *Journal of Gerontological Social Work*, *53*(3), 251–269. doi:10.1080/01634370903478989 PMID:20336572

Kiecolt-Glaser, J. K., Dura, J. R., Speicher, C. E., Trask, O. J., & Glaser, R. (1991). Spousal caregivers of dementia victims: Longitudinal changes in immunity and health. *Psychosomatic Medicine*, *53*(4), 345–362. doi:10.1097/00006842-199107000-00001 PMID:1656478

King, W. C., Belle, S. H., Brach, J. S., Simkin-Silverman, L. R., Soska, T., & Kriska, A. M. (2005). Objective measures of neighborhood environment and physical activity in older women. *American Journal of Preventive Medicine*, *28*(5), 461–469. doi:10.1016/j.amepre.2005.02.001 PMID:15894150

Kolhberg, L. (1973). The claim to moral adequacy of a highest stage of moral development. *Journal of Philosophy, 70*(18), 630-646.

Kramer, B., & Thompson, E. (Eds.). (2002). *Men as caregivers*. New York, NY: Springer Publishing Company.

Kramer, B. J. (1997). Gain in the caregiving experience: Where are we? What next? *The Gerontologist, 37*(2), 218–232. doi:10.1093/geront/37.2.218 PMID:9127978

Langford, P. E. (1995). *Essays in developmental psychology: Approaches to the development of moral reasoning*. Lawrence Erthbaum Associates Ltd. Press.

Logan Pearsall Smith. (n.d.). *AZQuotes.com*. Retrieved May 27, 2018, from AZQuotes.com Web site: http://www.azquotes.com/quote/556212

Losada, A., Pérez-Peñaranda, A., Rodriguez-Sanchez, E., Gomez-Marcos, M. A., Ballesteros-Rios, C., Ramos-Carrera, I. R., ... García-Ortiz, L. (2010). Leisure and distress in caregivers for elderly patients. *Archives of Gerontology and Geriatrics, 50*(3), 347–350. doi:10.1016/j.archger.2009.06.001 PMID:19573933

Maraboli, S. (2009). *Life, the truth & being free*. Port Washington, NY: Better Today Publishing.

Marsh, D. T., Lefley, H. P., Evans-Rhodes, D., Ansell, V. I., Doerzbacher, B. M., LaBarbera, L., & Paluzzi, J. E. (1996). The family experience of mental illness: Evidence for resilience. *Psychiatric Rehabilitation Journal, 20*(2), 3–12. doi:10.1037/h0095390

Matthews, D. A., & Clark, C. (1999). *The faith factor: Proof of the healing power of prayer*. New York, NY: Penguin.

McDaid, D. (2001). Estimating the costs of informal care for people with Alzheimer's disease: Methodological and practical challenges. *International Journal of Geriatric Psychiatry, 16*(4), 400–405. doi:10.1002/gps.353 PMID:11333428

Miller, B., Townsend, A., Carpenter, E., Montgomery, R. V., Stull, D., & Young, R. F. (2001). Social support and caregiver distress a replication analysis. *The Journals of Gerontology. Series B, Psychological Sciences and Social Sciences, 56*(4), S249–S256. doi:10.1093/geronb/56.4.S249 PMID:11445617

Moen, P., Robison, J., & Dempster-McClain, D. (1995). Caregiving and women's wellbeing: A life course approach. *Journal of Health and Social Behavior*, *36*(3), 259–273. doi:10.2307/2137342 PMID:7594358

Montgomery, C. L. (1991). The caregiving relationship: Paradoxical and transcendent aspects. *Journal of Transpersonal Psychology*, *23*, 91–104.

National Alliance for Caregiving. (2009, November). *Caregiving in the U.S.* Bethesda, MD: Author.

National Opinion Research Center. (2014, May). *Long term care in America: Expectations and realities*. Retrieved from http://www.longtermcarepoll.org/PDFs/LTC%202014/AP-NORC-Long-Term%20Care%20in%20America_FINAL%20WEB.pdf

Nicci, L. P. (1989). *Moral development and character education*. Berkeley, CA: Mrcuthrhan Publishing Corporation.

Nieboer, A. P., Schulz, R., Matthews, K. A., Scheier, M. F., Ormel, J., & Lindenberg, S. M. (1998). Spousal caregivers' activity restriction and depression: A model for changes over time. *Social Science & Medicine*, *47*(9), 1361–1371. doi:10.1016/S0277-9536(98)00214-7 PMID:9783879

Oishi, S., Kesebir, S., & Diener, E. (2011). Income inequality and happiness. *Psychological Science*, *22*(9), 1095–1100. doi:10.1177/0956797611417262 PMID:21841151

Pargament, K. I. (2010). Religion and coping: The current state of knowledge. In S. Folkman (Ed.), *The Oxford handbook of stress, health, and coping* (pp. 269–288). New York, NY: Oxford University Press. doi:10.1093/oxfordhb/9780195375343.013.0014

Payne, S., & Morbey, H. (2013). *Supporting family carers: Report on the evidence of how to work with and support family carers to inform the work of the Commission into the Future of Hospice Care*. Retrieved from http://eprints.lancs.ac.uk/68478/1/Supporting_family_carers.pdf

Pierre Teilhard de Chardin Quotes. (n.d.a). *BrainyQuote.com*. Retrieved May 27, 2018, from BrainyQuote.com Web site: https://www.brainyquote.com/quotes/pierre_teilhard_de_chardi_156693

Pierre Teilhard de Chardin Quotes. (n.d.b). *BrainyQuote.com*. Retrieved June 2, 2018, from BrainyQuote.com Web site: https://www.brainyquote.com/quotes/pierre_teilhard_de_chardi_156693

Poindexter, C. C., Linsk, N. L., & Warner, R. S. (1999). "He listens…Never gossip:" Spiritual coping without church support among older, predominantly African-American caregivers of persons with HIV. *Review of Religious Research*, *40*(3), 230–243. doi:10.2307/3512369

Porter, L. S., Keefe, F. J., Garst, J., McBride, C. M., & Baucom, D. (2008). Self-efficacy for managing pain, symptoms, and function in patients with lung cancer and their informal caregivers: Associations with symptoms and distress. *Pain*, *137*(2), 306–315. doi:10.1016/j.pain.2007.09.010 PMID:17942229

Power, F. C., Higgins, A., & Kohlberg, L. (1989). *Lawerence Kohlberg's approach to moral education*. New York: Columbia University Press.

Pressler, S. J., Gradus-Pizlo, I., Chubinski, S. D., Smith, G., Wheeler, S., Sloan, R., & Jung, M. (2013). Family caregivers of patients with heart failure: A longitudinal study. *The Journal of Cardiovascular Nursing*, *28*(5), 417–428. doi:10.1097/JCN.0b013e3182563877 PMID:22760173

Pressman, S. D., Matthews, K. A., Cohen, S., Martire, L. M., Scheier, M., Baum, A., & Schulz, R. (2009). Association of enjoyable leisure activities with psychological and physical wellbeing. *Psychosomatic Medicine*, *71*(7), 725–732. doi:10.1097/PSY.0b013e3181ad7978 PMID:19592515

Pruchno, R. A., Kleban, M. H., Michaels, J. E., & Dempsey, N. P. (1990). Mental and physical health of caregiving spouses: Development of a causal model. *Journal of Gerontology*, *45*(5), 192–P199. doi:10.1093/geronj/45.5.P192 PMID:2394915

Rabinowitz, Y. G., Mausbach, B. T., & Gallagher-Thompson, D. (2009). Self-efficacy as a moderator of the relationship between care recipient memory and behavioral problems and caregiver depression in female dementia caregivers. *Alzheimer Disease and Associated Disorders*, *23*(4), 389–394. doi:10.1097/WAD.0b013e3181b6f74d PMID:19935146

Rapp, S. R., Shumaker, S., Schmidt, S., Naughton, M., & Anderson, R. (1998). Social resourcefulness: Its relationship to social support and wellbeing among caregivers of dementia victims. *Aging & Mental Health*, *2*(1), 40–48. doi:10.1080/13607869856920

Redinbaugh, E. M., MacCallum, R. C., & Kiecolt-Glaser, J. K. (1995). Recurrent syndromal depression in caregivers. *Psychology and Aging*, *10*(3), 358–368. doi:10.1037/0882-7974.10.3.358 PMID:8527057

Rivera, P. A., Rose, J. M., Futterman, A., Lovett, S. B., & Gallagher-Thompson, D. (1991). Dimensions of perceived social support in clinically depressed and nondepressed female caregivers. *Psychology and Aging*, *6*(2), 232–237. doi:10.1037/0882-7974.6.2.232 PMID:1863392

Roberts, H., Halpin-Healy, C., McGinnis, R., & Noble, J. (2014). Museum-based creative arts programming is associated with less dementia patient apathy and better caregiver wellbeing. *Neurology*, *82*(10Supplement), 1–002.

Robinson, B. (1983). Validation of a caregiver strain index. *Journal of Gerontology*, *38*(3), 344–348. doi:10.1093/geronj/38.3.344 PMID:6841931

Rodríguez-Sánchez, E., Pérez-Peñaranda, A., Losada-Baltar, A., Pérez-Arechaederra, D., Gómez-Marcos, M. Á., Patino-Alonso, M. C., & García-Ortiz, L. (2011). Relationships between quality of life and family function in caregiver. *BMC Family Practice*, *12*(1), 1. doi:10.1186/1471-2296-12-19 PMID:21496270

Romero-Moreno, R., Losada, A., Mausbach, B. T., Márquez-González, M., Patterson, T. L., & López, J. (2011). Analysis of the moderating effect of self-efficacy domains in different points of the dementia caregiving process. *Aging & Mental Health*, *15*(2), 221–231. doi:10.1080/13607863.2010.505231 PMID:20924819

Ross, L., Holliman, D., & Dixon, D. R. (2003). Resiliency in family caregivers: Implications for social work practice. *Journal of Gerontological Social Work*, *40*(3), 81–96. doi:10.1300/J083v40n03_07

Scharlach, A. E. (1994). Caregiving and employment: Competing or complementary roles? *The Gerontologist*, *34*(3), 378–385. doi:10.1093/geront/34.3.378 PMID:8076880

Schryer, E., Mock, S. E., Hilbrecht, M., Lero, D., & Smale, B. (2016). Use of leisure facilities and wellbeing of adult caregivers. *Leisure Sciences*, *38*(1), 17–33. doi:10.1080/01490400.2015.1038373

Schüz, B., Czerniawski, A., Davie, N., Miller, L., Quinn, M. G., King, C., ... Scott, J. L. (2015). Leisure time activities and mental health in informal dementia caregivers. *Applied Psychology. Health and Wellbeing*, *7*(2), 230–248. doi:10.1111/aphw.12046 PMID:26097155

Schwarzer, R., Dunkel-Schetter, C., & Kemeny, M. (1994). The multidimensional nature of received social support in gay men at risk of HIV infection and AIDS. *American Journal of Community Psychology*, *22*(3), 319–339. doi:10.1007/BF02506869 PMID:7879745

Schwarzer, R., & Jerusalem, M. (1995). Generalized Self-Efficacy Scale. In J. Weinman, S. Wright, & M. Johnston (Eds.), *Measures in health psychology: A user's portfolio. Causal and control beliefs* (pp. 35–37). Windsor, UK: NFER-Nelson.

Shenk, D. (2014). *Someone to lend a helping hand: Women growing old in rural America* (Vol. 13). New York, NY: Routledge.

Silliman, R. A. (1993). Predictors of family caregivers' physical and psychological health following hospitalization of their elders. *Journal of the American Geriatrics Society*, *41*(10), 1039–1046. doi:10.1111/j.1532-5415.1993.tb06450.x PMID:8409148

Sisk, R. J. (2000). Caregiver burden and health promotion. *International Journal of Nursing Studies*, *37*(1), 37–43. doi:10.1016/S0020-7489(99)00053-X PMID:10687808

Smith, B. W., Dalen, J., Wiggins, K., Tooley, E., Christopher, P., & Bernard, J. (2008). The Brief Resilience Scale: Assessing the ability to bounce back. *International Journal of Behavioral Medicine*, *15*(3), 194–200. doi:10.1080/10705500802222972 PMID:18696313

Speers, P., & Walker, T. (2013). *The inspired caregiver: finding joy while caring for those you love*. Seattle, WA: Createspace Independent Publishing Platform.

Staight, P. R., & Harvey, S. M. (1990). Caregiver burden: A comparison between elderly women as primary and secondary caregivers for their spouses. *Journal of Gerontological Social Work*, *15*(1-2), 89–104. doi:10.1300/J083v15n01_10

Stevens, A. B., Coon, D., Wisniewski, S., Vance, D., Arguelles, S., Belle, S., ... Ory, M. (2004). Measurement of leisure time satisfaction in family caregivers. *Aging & Mental Health*, *8*(5), 450–459. doi:10.1080/13607860410001709737 PMID:15511743

Stone, R. I., & Short, P. F. (1990). The competing demands of employment and informal caregiving to disabled elders. *Medical Care*, *28*(6), 513–526. doi:10.1097/00005650-199006000-00004 PMID:2355757

Taylor, E. J. (2006, July). Prevalence and associated factors of spiritual needs among patients with cancer and family caregivers. *Oncology Nursing Forum*, *33*(4), 729–735. doi:10.1188/06.ONF.729-735 PMID:16858453

Thompson, E. H., Futterman, A. M., Gallagher-Thompson, D., Rose, J. M., & Lovett, S. B. (1993). Social support and caregiving burden in family caregivers of frail elders. *Journal of Gerontology*, *48*(5), S245–S254. doi:10.1093/geronj/48.5.S245 PMID:8366273

Thorsteinsson, E. B., & James, J. E. (1999). A meta-analysis of the effects of experimental manipulations of social support during laboratory stress. *Psychology & Health*, *14*(5), 869–886. doi:10.1080/08870449908407353

Toseland, R. W., McCallion, P., Gerber, T., & Banks, S. (2002). Predictors of health and human services use by persons with dementia and their family caregivers. *Social Science & Medicine*, *55*(7), 1255–1266. doi:10.1016/S0277-9536(01)00240-4 PMID:12365535

Tuck, I. (2004). Development of a spirituality intervention to promote healing. *Journal of Theory Construction & Testing*, *8*(2).

Uchino, B. N. (2009). Understanding the links between social support and physical health: A life-span perspective with emphasis on the separability of perceived and received support. *Perspectives on Psychological Science*, *4*(3), 236–255. doi:10.1111/j.1745-6924.2009.01122.x PMID:26158961

Unger, D. G., & Powell, D. R. (1980). Supporting families under stress: The role of social networks. *Family Relations*, *29*(4), 566–574. doi:10.2307/584473

Uno, D., Uchino, B. N., & Smith, T. W. (2002). Relationship quality moderates the effect of social support given by close friends on cardiovascular reactivity in women. *International Journal of Behavioral Medicine*, *9*(3), 243–262. doi:10.1207/S15327558IJBM0903_06 PMID:12360840

van den Berg, B., Fiebig, D. G., & Hall, J. (2014). Wellbeing losses due to care-giving. *Journal of Health Economics*, *35*(100), 123–131. doi:10.1016/j.jhealeco.2014.01.008 PMID:24662888

van den Berg, J. W., Geertsma, A., van der Bij, W. I. M., Koeter, G. H., de Boer, W. J., Postma, D. S., & ten Vergert, E. M. (2000). Bronchiolitis obliterans syndrome after lung transplantation and health-related quality of life. *American Journal of Respiratory and Critical Care Medicine*, *161*(6), 1937–1941. doi:10.1164/ajrccm.161.6.9909092 PMID:10852770

Wakui, T., Saito, T., Agree, E. M., & Kai, I. (2012). Effects of home, outside leisure, social, and peer activity on psychological health among Japanese family caregivers. *Aging & Mental Health*, *16*(4), 500–506. doi:10.1080/13607863.2011.644263 PMID:22360698

Waldron, S. (2010). *Measuring subjective wellbeing in the UK* (ONS working paper). Retrieved from http://www.ons.gov.uk/ons/guide-method/user-guidance/wellbeing/publications/measuring-subjective-wellbeing-in-the-uk.pdf

Washington, M. (n.d.). *Letter, Martha Washington to Mercy Otis Warren, December 26, 1789*. Martha Washington, Item #25. Retrieved from http://marthawashington.us/items/show/25

Watkins, T. (2014). Decreasing informal caregiver burden with social media. *Home Healthcare Now*, *32*(5), 304–308. doi:10.1097/NHH.0000000000000058 PMID:24802601

Welch, D. C., & West, R. L. (1995). Self-efficacy and mastery: Its application to issues of environmental control, cognition, and aging. *Developmental Review*, *15*(2), 150–171. doi:10.1006/drev.1995.1007

Werner, E. E., & Smith, R. S. (2001). *Journeys from childhood to midlife: Risk, resilience, and recovery*. Ithaca, NY: Cornell University Press.

White-Means, S. I., & Chang, C. F. (1994). Informal caregivers' leisure time and stress. *Journal of Family and Economic Issues*, *15*(2), 117–136. doi:10.1007/BF02353636

Wilks, S. E., & Croom, B. (2008). Perceived stress and resilience in Alzheimer's disease caregivers: Testing moderation and mediation models of social support. *Aging & Mental Health*, *12*(3), 357–365. doi:10.1080/13607860801933323 PMID:18728949

Williams, S. W., & Dilworth-Anderson, P. (2002). Systems of social support in families who care for dependent African American elders. *The Gerontologist*, *42*(2), 224–236. doi:10.1093/geront/42.2.224 PMID:11914466

Williams, S. W., Williams, C. S., Zimmerman, S., Munn, J., Dobbs, D., & Sloane, P. D. (2008). Emotional and physical health of informal caregivers of residents at the end of life: The role of social support. *The Journals of Gerontology. Series B, Psychological Sciences and Social Sciences*, *63*(3), S171–S183. doi:10.1093/geronb/63.3.S171 PMID:18559692

Williamson, G. M., Shaffer, D. R., & Schulz, R. (1998). Activity restriction and prior relationship history as contributors to mental health outcomes among middle-aged and older spousal caregivers. *Health Psychology*, *17*(2), 152–162. doi:10.1037/0278-6133.17.2.152 PMID:9548706

Wilson, W. R. (1967). Correlates of avowed happiness. *Psychological Bulletin*, *67*(4), 294–306. doi:10.1037/h0024431 PMID:6042458

Yang, S. J., & Chen, I. Y. (2008). A social network-based system for supporting interactive collaboration in knowledge sharing over peer-to-peer network. *International Journal of Human-Computer Studies*, *66*(1), 36–50. doi:10.1016/j.ijhcs.2007.08.005

Yates, M. E., Tennstedt, S., & Chang, B. (1999). Contributors to and mediators of psychological wellbeing for informal caregivers. *The Journals of Gerontology. Series B, Psychological Sciences and Social Sciences*, *54B*(1), S12–S22. doi:10.1093/geronb/54B.1.P12 PMID:9934391

Yee, J. L., & Schulz, R. (2000). Gender differences in psychiatric morbidity among family caregivers: A review and analysis. *The Gerontologist*, *40*(2), 147–164. doi:10.1093/geront/40.2.147 PMID:10820918

Zarit, S. H., Reever, K. E., & Bach-Peterson, J. (1980). Relatives of the impaired elderly: Correlates of feelings of burden. *The Gerontologist*, *20*(6), 649–655. doi:10.1093/geront/20.6.649 PMID:7203086

Zeiss, A. M., Gallagher-Thompson, D., Lovett, S., Rose, J., & McKibbin, C. (1999). Self-efficacy as a mediator of caregiver coping: Development and testing of an assessment model. *Journal of Clinical Geropsychology*, *5*(3), 221–230. doi:10.1023/A:1022955817074

Zimet, G. D., Dahlem, N. W., Zimet, S. G., & Farley, G. K. (1988). The Multidimensional Scale of Perceived Social Support. *Journal of Personality Assessment*, *52*(1), 30–41. doi:10.120715327752jpa5201_2 PMID:2280326

ADDITIONAL READING

Kohlberg, L., Levine, C., & Hewer, A. (1983). *Moral stages: A current formulation and a response to critics*. Basel, NY: Karger.

Lambrozo, T. (2009). The role of moral commitments in moral judgment. *Cognitive Science Society*, *33*(2), 273–286. doi:10.1111/j.1551-6709.2009.01013.x PMID:21585471

Munhall, F. (1980). Moral reason levels of nursing students. *Image*, *12*(3), 18–31. doi:10.1111/j.1547-5069.1980.tb01467.x PMID:11653753

Singer, P. (1993). *A companion to ethics*. Oxford, UK: Blackwell Publishers and New Malden.

Chapter 2
Methodological and Conceptual Approach

ABSTRACT

This chapter presents the methodological and conceptual approach, which informed the research design for the study. It is pertinent to reiterate here that the design of this study sought to discern the positive psychological forces that shape subjective wellbeing of informal caregivers. This desire prompted the adoption of a mixed methods research. The rationale for this methodological preference is presented. In addition, advantages of mixed methods approach are elaborated upon. Furthermore, other issues are addressed, including sample size, instrumentation, and research procedures. This chapter also explains, with much detail, the parameters and boundary conditions that constituted the guiding assumptions, limitations, as well as delimitations of the study. It should be noted that the chapter also explains the essential approach to data analysis.

INTRODUCTION

This chapter commences with a restatement of the primary purpose of this study and the problem as explained in the Introduction. As referred to above, it includes details of the theoretical framework used to test the influence of self-efficacy, spirituality, social support, resilience, and participation in leisure activities on the subjective wellbeing of informal caregivers. Also explained is the use of a concurrent mixed methods research design, including

DOI: 10.4018/978-1-5225-7452-1.ch002

the sample selection, sample size, selection of participants, instrumentation, methodological assumptions, procedures, limitations, data collection methods, and data analysis.

The Introduction contained evidence of the vast disparity of research regarding the positive aspects of caregiving. Informal caregivers as well as the communities offering them support (e.g., advocacy groups, medical institutions, social service agencies, religious organizations, and the general populace) seek guidance, direction, and resources in managing the concerns surrounding wellbeing that arise for the caregiver. As alluded to earlier, a vast majority of the existing literature focused on the negative aspects of the caregiving experience, indicating caregiving is harmful to physical health (Pruchno et al., 1990) and can affect participation in detrimental indulgences such as excessive alcohol consumption, binge eating, and smoking (Gallant & Connell, 1998). There is limited research regarding the positive aspects of informal caregiving (Boerner et al., 2004), yet claims exist emphasizing that the informal caregiver experience can be rewarding for both the caregiver and care recipient. It may also provide a sense of belonging and purpose, and can be uplifting to the informal caregiver (Boerner et al., 2004; Kramer, 1997).

In Chapter 1, the researcher discussed the theoretical framework of the study— subjective wellbeing—which also served as the dependent variable. Additionally, the independent variables of self-efficacy, social support, resilience, spirituality, and leisure participation were discussed in relation to the study's stipulated hypotheses.

PURPOSE AND RATIONALE OF MIXED METHODS RESEARCH

The purpose of this study was to methodically examine the factors of self-efficacy, spirituality, social support, resilience, and leisure participation and their influence on the subjective wellbeing of informal caregivers. In carrying out its function in this manner, the chapter provides a description of the methods employed to conduct the research. Thus according to Creswell (2009), in the selection of a research design, the researcher's decision should be based on the worldview and assumptions the researcher brings to the study, procedures of inquiry, and specific methods of data collection, analysis, and interpretation (p. 3). Zoellner (2017, p.683) defines mixed methods research as follows: "It explores phenomena utilizing a combination of QUAL and QUAN methods in a single inquiry to gain more complete perspective." Zoellner (p.683) also considers mixed methods research the third research paradigm in addition to quantitative and qualitative research. In explaining the rationale for mixed methods research, Griensven, Moore and Hall (2014, p.308) intimate that mixed methods research "may be viewed as providing a complete and deeper understanding of the subject under investigation." Zoellner (2017, p. 686) identified six mixed methods research designs to address research problems. They are as follows: 1) convergent parallel, 2) explanatory sequential, 3) exploratory sequential, 4) embedded, 5) transformative, and 6) multiphase.

Some scholars have suggested that mixed methods research tend to give prominence to quantitative methods and relegate qualitative methods to an auxiliary position (p.370). It is reported that this may be a consequence, in part, of the demands of service users, governments and funders (p. 370). Freshwater (2007) contends that mixed methods research offers contexts for methodological criticism. However, concurring with Morse (1991), we argue that one of the advantages of a mixed methods study is that it enables the researcher to collect data at the same time (concurrent or parallel design) or to collect data at different points (sequential or two-stage designs).

In line with the requirements of mixed methods research, the instrument distributed to each participant in this study had both quantitative and qualitative questions. According to Mays and Pope (1995), the objective of qualitative research is the expansion of thoughts that explain social phenomena in their natural setting, putting the emphasis on the participants of the research. Hence, the open-ended questions in the survey used in the current study were developed as a means to gain additional insight into the respondents' perceptions. The quantitative component of the study involved the use of correlation and multiple regression statistical methods to measure the responses of the participants. The researchers then analyzed the data for patterns, similarities and differences.

The findings of the study contribute to research into critical factors that may influence the wellbeing of the informal caregiver. In order for the objectives of the study to be realized, it was anchored around five research hypotheses. Readers would note that the research question and hypotheses are presented above in the preface. This chapter concludes with the methodological assumptions and limitations inherent in the study.

RESEARCH DESIGN

The purpose of this study was to examine the impact of various variables on the subjective wellbeing of informal caregivers. A concurrent mixed methods research design was used in the study. A further critical benefit of a mixed methods study is the capacity to enable the researcher to collect data at the same time (Morse, 1991). Thus, the instrument used a combination of quantitative measurement scales with qualitative open-ended questions. The reason for the application of this design was that it provided a well-rounded approach to assessing the views of the population under study.

A visual rendering of the research design is depicted in Figure 1.

Sample Selection and Size

Two churches located in Chicago, Illinois, were selected because they had large populations of congregants. Additionally, the majority of the membership base had been with the church for generations.

Figure 1. Concurrent mixed methods design visual depiction

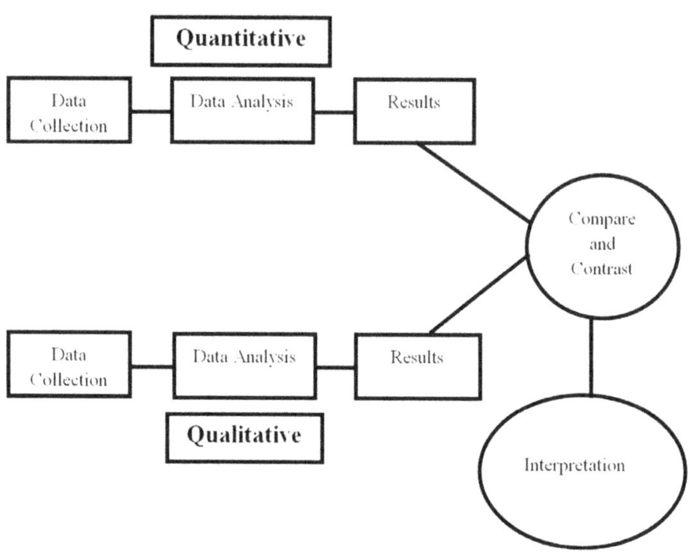

Instrumentation

The independent variable of subjective wellbeing was measured with the Personal Wellbeing Index (PWI-A; International Wellbeing Group, 2013), which consists of eight questions.

The dependent variables were measured with the following scales:

- Self-efficacy was measured with the General Self-Efficacy Scale (Schwarzer & Jerusalem, 1995), which consists of 10 items.
- Social support was measured with the Multidimensional Scale of Perceived Social Support (MSPSS; Zimet, Dahlem, Zimet, & Farley, 1988), which consists of 12 items.
- Spirituality was measured with the Intrinsic Spirituality Scale (Hodge, 2003), which consists of six items.
- Leisure participation was measured with the Leisure Time Satisfaction Scale (Stevens et al., 2004), which consists of six items.
- Resilience was measured with the Resilience scale (Smith et al., 2008), which consists of six items.

Procedures

On consecutive Sundays during the months of February and March of 2016, the pastors from two churches allowed the researchers to present before the congregants to inform them of their study and its significance to the informal caregiver population. The researchers asked congregants who identified as informal caregivers to meet with them in an adjacent room. These individuals were then separately and discreetly asked pre-screening questions (See Appendix A). If they qualified based on their responses, they were then handed a consent form and survey (See Appendix B) to peruse, sign, and then answer. Those individuals who had time completed the survey immediately, while others were allowed to take the survey home and return it the following Sunday. The survey collection period lasted 8 weeks. All participants were between the ages of 18 and 80 years. There were 26 females and 10 males, for a total of 36 participants. All identified as African American.

METHODOLOGICAL ASSUMPTIONS, LIMITATIONS, AND DELIMITATIONS

Methodological Assumptions

The current study involved a mixed methods research design that was grounded in several methodological assumptions:

- The participants were actual informal caregivers.
- The answers provided by the participants in this study (informal caregivers) were reflective of their truth and they gave careful consideration regarding the information requested.
- The survey instrument created for this study was applicable for the design of the study and the purpose for which it was employed.
- The researchers' influence on the data collected and recorded was insignificant and need not be considered in the study.

Limitations

The data gathered in this investigation were limited by the scope and design of this study. For this reason, the study was limited as follows:

- The instrument was a self-report questionnaire and responses could possibly vary under different emotional conditions of the participants.
- Truthfulness of the responses may be questionable because of the sensitivity of the topic.
- The study reflected the experiences and opinions of a small number of informal caregivers and therefore results may not be able to be generalized to the overall population.

Delimitations

For the current research study, definite limits pertaining to collecting, compiling, and interpreting results were established. For this reason, this study was delimited as follows:

- The study participants consisted of informal caregivers only.
- The choice of sample size may have seriously affected the findings considering that not 100% of the population was used.
- The study involved the use of a purposive sampling technique; therefore, the results obtained may not allow for a more complete representation of the populous.

DATA ANALYSIS

The information obtained from the survey instrument was analyzed and categorized into meaningful groups. For instance, the insights gathered from the quantitative instruments were assessed via SPSS (Statistical Package for the Social Sciences). This software consists of an integrated series of computer programs that enable a researcher to read data from surveys and manipulate them in various ways to produce a wide range of statistical analyses and reports together with documentation. The data points entered were statistically analyzed and conclusions were produced. The quantitative analysis included descriptive statistics as well as inferential statistical analysis. The qualitative segment was summarized according to the systematic process suggested by Creswell (2007) that involves analyzing qualitative data using a coding system. This system is delineated in the following categories:

- Codes on topics that readers expect to find based on past literature and common sense.
- Codes that are surprising and that were not anticipated at the beginning of the study.
- Codes that are unusual and that are, in and of themselves, of conceptual interest to readers.
- Codes that address a larger theoretical perspective in the research (Creswell, 2007).

Propositions or conclusions were finally drawn after integrating the information received via the qualitative and quantitative portions of the study.

VALIDITY AND RELIABILITY

Validity is often considered to be the most important property of an assessment tool. Considerable time was devoted to making certain the items on the survey were clearly worded, well defined, and had high face and content validity. *Reliability* is the degree to which a set of items consistently measures the same thing across respondents and institutional settings (Creswell, 2007; Mengshoel, 2012). The surveys used in this study each had been previously tested to ensure that both the components of validity and reliability were strong (Creswell, 2007; Creswell, 2009).

CONCLUSION

Chapter 2 contained a restatement of the purpose of the study and why a concurrent mixed methods triangulation approach was used for this study. According to Leedy and Ormond (2005), the type of research design chosen for a specific research problem should consider the type of data to be collected in the unraveling of the problem. This study was conducted at two churches in Illinois. Over a 2-month period (February and March of 2016), pre-screening questionnaires and surveys were distributed to congregants at these churches who identified as informal caregivers. The researchers sought to determine the significant factors that contribute to the subjective wellbeing of informal caregivers via the use of a survey that contained closed- and open-ended questions. The data generated from this instrument and analysis of the results are presented in the next. Readers will note that analysis of data presented in the next chapter sought to address issues as they relate to the pertinent and therefore stipulated research question and hypotheses in this study.

REFERENCES

Boerner, K., Schulz, R., & Horowitz, A. (2004). Positive aspects of caregiving and adaptation to bereavement. *Psychology and Aging*, *19*(4), 668–675. doi:10.1037/0882-7974.19.4.668 PMID:15584791

Cameron, R., Sankaran, S., & Scales, J. (2015). Mixed method use in project management research. *Project Management Journal*, *46*(2), 90–104. doi:10.1002/pmj.21484

Creswell, J. W. (2007). *Qualitative inquiry and research design: Choosing among five approaches* (2nd ed.). Thousand Oaks, CA: Sage.

Creswell, J. W. (2009). *Research design: Qualitative, quantitative, and mixed methods approaches* (3rd ed.). Los Angeles, CA: Sage Publications.

Freshwater, D. (2007). Reading mixed methods research: Contexts for criticism. *Journal of Mixed Methods Research*, *1*(2), 134–146. doi:10.1177/1558689806298578

Gallant, M. P., & Connell, C. M. (1998). The stress process among dementia spouse caregivers: Are caregivers at risk for negative health behavior change? *Research on Aging*, *20*(3), 267–297. doi:10.1177/0164027598203001

Griensven, H. V., Moore, A. P., & Hall, V. (2014). The best of both worlds? *Manual Therapy*, *19*(5), 367–371. doi:10.1016/j.math.2014.05.005 PMID:24924515

Hodge, D. R. (2003). The Intrinsic Spirituality Scale: A new six-item instrument for assessing the salience of spirituality as a motivational construct. *Journal of Social Service Research*, *30*(1), 41–61. doi:10.1300/J079v30n01_03

International Wellbeing Group. (2013). *Personal Wellbeing Index* (5th ed.). Melbourne, Australia: Australian Centre on Quality of Life, Deakin University. Retrieved from http://www.deakin.edu.au/research/acqol/instruments/well-being-index/index.php

Kramer, B. J. (1997). Gain in the caregiving experience: Where are we? What next? *The Gerontologist*, *37*(2), 218–232. doi:10.1093/geront/37.2.218 PMID:9127978

Leedy, P. D., & Ormond, J. E. (2005). *Practical research: Planning and design*. Essex, UK: Pearson.

Mays, N., & Pope, C. (1995). Rigour and qualitative research. *BMJ: British Medical Journal*, *311*(6997), 109–112. doi:10.1136/bmj.311.6997.109 PMID:7613363

Mengshoel, A. M. (2012). Mixed methods research: So far easier said than done? *Manual Therapy*, *17*(4), 373–375. doi:10.1016/j.math.2012.02.006 PMID:22405885

Morse, J. M. (1991). Approaches to qualitative-quantitative methodological triangulation. *Nursing Research*, *40*(2), 120–123. doi:10.1097/00006199-199103000-00014 PMID:2003072

Pruchno, R. A., Kleban, M. H., Michaels, J. E., & Dempsey, N. P. (1990). Mental and physical health of caregiving spouses: Development of a causal model. *Journal of Gerontology*, *45*(5), 192–P199. doi:10.1093/geronj/45.5.P192 PMID:2394915

Schwarzer, R., & Jerusalem, M. (1995). Generalized Self-Efficacy Scale. In J. Weinman, S. Wright, & M. Johnston (Eds.), *Measures in health psychology: A user's portfolio. Causal and control beliefs* (pp. 35–37). Windsor, UK: NFER-Nelson.

Smith, B. W., Dalen, J., Wiggins, K., Tooley, E., Christopher, P., & Bernard, J. (2008). The Brief Resilience Scale: Assessing the ability to bounce back. *International Journal of Behavioral Medicine*, *15*(3), 194–200. doi:10.1080/10705500802222972 PMID:18696313

Stevens, A. B., Coon, D., Wisniewski, S., Vance, D., Arguelles, S., Belle, S., ... Ory, M. (2004). Measurement of leisure time satisfaction in family caregivers. *Aging & Mental Health*, *8*(5), 450–459. doi:10.1080/13607860410001709737 PMID:15511743

Zimet, G. D., Dahlem, N. W., Zimet, S. G., & Farley, G. K. (1988). The Multidimensional Scale of Perceived Social Support. *Journal of Personality Assessment*, *52*(1), 30–41. doi:10.120715327752jpa5201_2 PMID:2280326

Zoellner, J., & Harris, J. E. (2017). Mixed methods research in nutrition and dietetics. *Journal of the Academy of Nutrition and Dietetics*, *17*(5), 683–697. doi:10.1016/j.jand.2017.01.018 PMID:28284525

ADDITIONAL READING

Greene, J. C. (2008). Is mixed methods social inquiry a distinctive methodology? *Journal of Mixed Methods Research*, *2*(1), 7–22. doi:10.1177/1558689807309969

Johnson, B. R., & Onwuegbuzie, A. J. (2004). Mixed methods research: A research paradigm whose time has come. *Educational Researcher*, *33*(7), 14–26. doi:10.3102/0013189X033007014

Johnson, B. R., Onwuegbuzie, A. J., & Turner, L. A. (2007). Toward a definition of mixed methods research. *Journal of Mixed Methods Research*, *1*(1), 112–133. doi:10.1177/1558689806298224

Leech, N., & Onwuegbuzie, A. J. (2009). A typology of mixed methods research designs. *Quality & Quantity*, *43*(2), 265–275. doi:10.100711135-007-9105-3

Sale, J. E., Lohfeld, L. H., & Brazil, K. (2002). Revisiting the quantitative –qualitative debate: Implications for mixed methods research. *Quality & Quantity*, *36*(1), 43–53. doi:10.1023/A:1014301607592 PMID:26523073

Chapter 3
Presentation of Research Findings

ABSTRACT

Most of the research participants believed their caregiving responsibilities adversely affected their subjective wellbeing. Some of the research participants believed their caregiving responsibilities had a positive psychological effect on their subjective wellbeing. Meanwhile, a significant number of research participants believed they were innately capable of handling their caregiving responsibilities. Research participants had the perception that their spiritual beliefs were positively influential to their caregiver roles and their subjective wellbeing. Research participants seemed to rely on their spiritual convictions as the lynchpin in sustaining themselves in their roles as informal caregivers as it related to their subjective wellbeing. The variable family support was a significant factor. Similarly, the vast majority of research participants believed their resilience allowed them to be optimistic about their performance as caregivers. A significant number of the research participants believed they had limited time for leisure activities but felt this did not negatively affect their performance as informal caregivers.

DOI: 10.4018/978-1-5225-7452-1.ch003

INTRODUCTION

The Introduction and the first two chapters of this dissertation contained an explanation of the research problem and a concise review of the literature relevant to the subject of this study, as well as the research methodology that guided the current study. As previously stated, we relied on a mixed methods approach was adopted to facilitate the data analyses. The aim of this approach was to provide a thoroughly encompassing explanation of the research problem. This chapter provides the complete results of the data analyses conducted by the researchers to complete the research study's purpose through responding to the research question and hypotheses.

RESTATEMENT OF THE RESEARCH PURPOSE

The purpose of this mixed methods study was to examine how the variables of self-efficacy, spirituality, social support, resilience, and leisure participation influenced the subjective wellbeing of informal caregivers. The notion of how to enhance the subjective wellbeing of informal caregivers has garnered sufficient attention recently as the need for home-based care has increased exponentially. Notwithstanding this claim, it is paramount that further exploration of the aforementioned factors be supported by leaders of caregiving organizations, the medical community, researchers, and the general populace in the hopes that informal caregivers become more aware of influences central for them to maintain or enhance the quality of their lives during their tenure as caregivers.

Self-efficacy, in its purest sense, is a person's own belief that he or she can accomplish a specific goal or task. This concept holds much significance to informal caregivers as they encounter the challenges and triumphs associated with their position. It is germane to understand how informal caregivers' levels of self-efficacy evolve as they embrace their role.

Social support research pertaining to the informal caregiver has revealed various factors that make it of essential significance to a caregiver's wellbeing. A better understanding of its relevance to caregivers is of critical significance and was examined in this study.

Resilience, for the purpose of this study, was defined as the "positive or successful adaption, competence and functioning in the face of stressful experiences" (Gaugler et al., 2007, p. 38). Early researchers on resilience mainly explored the resilience levels of children in adverse settings. However, over the last few decades, researchers have also been examining how resilience affects caregivers and their abilities to manage individuals with chronic illnesses. The current study was designed to determine whether this concept has similar relevancy for the informal caregiver.

The influence of spirituality among the informal caregiver population is frequently credited as a dominantly positive element in helping them elevate their wellbeing and allowing them to put their caregiving role in perspective (Buck, 2006). This variable was included in the current study as the participants were members from two religious institutions.

Last, participation in leisure activities can help caregivers attain additional skills and knowledge, nurture social relationships, embrace positive emotions, and improve their quality of life (Wakui et al., 2012). This study was designed to distinguish whether participation in varied leisure activities could contribute to better subjective wellbeing for informal caregivers.

PROCEDURES

The researcher administered a survey consisting of 56 quantitative questions and six open-ended questions to informal caregivers living within the state of Illinois. Additionally, contained in the survey were questions related to the participants' demographics. Regression and correlation analysis were the principal methods of analysis. Given the limited sample size (n=36) and hence the non-parametric nature of the dataset, Spearman's *rho* based non-parametric correlations were calculated. However, the results did not show significant differences from the parametric correlations' results reported here. Stepwise regression with backward elimination was also employed to identify variables in the model that had the most impact on the dependent variable (Verma, 2013; Pallent, 2013; Salkind, 2016). Five hypotheses were stipulated that reflected attempts at a systematic analysis of the effects of the independent variables on the dependent variable (Onwuegbuzie & Teddie, 2003).

DESCRIPTIVE STATISTICS

This section presents descriptive statistics for the continuous and categorical variables in the study and the responses of the research participants. The variables presented were taken from the demographic section of the survey instrument (See Table 1).

Table 1 shows that a total of 36 individuals participated in the survey. The average age of the population sampled was between 46 and 55 years with a range from 18 to 75 and above. The research participants provided care to the care recipients from a minimum of 1 hour to a maximum of 12 hours or more per week. The number of months that the caregivers provided care to the care recipient ranged from a minimum of 2 to a maximum of 240.

Table 2 depicts the descriptive statistics for the dependent and independent variables. The table shows there was one dependent variable (i.e., subjective wellbeing) and five independent variables: self-efficacy, social support, resilience, spirituality, and leisure participation.

Table 3 shows the descriptive statistics for categorical variables such as gender, race, and caregiver relationships. A frequency analysis depicted that males comprised 28% of the participants and females comprised 72%. All of the participants identified their race as African American. Further frequency

Table 1.Descriptive Statistics for Control Variables for Survey Respondents (N = 36)

	Minimum	Maximum	*M*	*SD*
Age	1.0	6.0	3.194	1.117
Hours	1.0	5.0	4.028	1.082
Months	2.0	240	59.444	55.759
Gross Income	1.0	6.0	3.222	1.149

Table 2 .Descriptive Statistics for Dependent and Independent Variables (N = 36)

Variables	Minimum	Maximum	*M*	*SD*
Subjective Wellbeing	3.9	9.5	7.358	1.215
Self-Efficacy	2.6	4.9	4.033	.456
Social Support	2.8	5.0	3.880	.498
Resilience	2.5	3.7	3.009	.273
Spirituality	.0	10.0	8.157	2.028
Leisure Participation	1.3	2.0	1.306	.469

Table 3.Descriptive Statistics for Categorical Variables

Frequency Analysis	Gender		Race	Caregiver Relationship to Care Recipient			
	Male	Female	Black	Children/Grandchildren	Multiple	Parent	Spouse
	28%	72%	100%	5.6% 2.8%	25%	55.6%	11%

analysis of the caregiver relationships reflected that 55.6% of the participants cared for an ailing parent. Next to those who cared for ailing parents were those who cared for multiple individuals, constituting 25% of the sample. Those caring for spouses constituted 11% of the study participants. Individuals caring for children constituted 5.6% while those caring for grandchildren constituted 2.8% of the sample.

RESEARCH QUESTION AND HYPOTHESES TESTING

This section lists the research question and hypotheses of the study. As stated in the Introduction, there was one primary research question and five hypotheses formulated for the study. The research question that directed this study was as follows: What are the significant factors that contribute to increased levels of subjective wellbeing of informal caregivers?

Analysis of the Quantitative Data

The research question was addressed through the five sets of null and alternative hypotheses:

- **$H1_0$:** There is no relationship between self-efficacy and the subjective wellbeing of informal caregivers.
- **$H1_a$:** There is a positive relationship between self-efficacy and the subjective wellbeing of informal caregivers.
- **$H2_0$:** There is no relationship between social support and the subjective wellbeing of informal caregivers.
- **$H2_a$:** There is a positive relationship between social support and the subjective wellbeing of informal caregivers.
- **$H3_0$:** There is no relationship between resilience and the subjective wellbeing of informal caregivers.

- **H3$_a$:** There is a positive relationship between resilience and the subjective wellbeing of informal caregivers.
- **H4$_0$:** There is no relationship between spirituality and the subjective wellbeing of informal caregivers.
- **H4$_a$:** There is a positive relationship between spirituality and the subjective wellbeing of informal caregivers.
- **H5$_0$:** There is no relationship between leisure participation and the subjective wellbeing of informal caregivers.
- **H5$_a$:** There is a positive relationship between leisure participation and the subjective wellbeing of informal caregivers.

The results of the correlation analysis in Table 4 show there was no statistically significant relationship between age and subjective wellbeing (r = .118, p = .492). The results also showed there was no statistically significant relationship between gender and subjective wellbeing (r = .043, p = .804). Next, there was no statistically significant relationship between gross income and subjective wellbeing (r = .192, p = .262). The results also showed there was a statistically significant relationship between the number of months that an informal caregiver provided care to a care recipient and the subjective wellbeing of that informal caregiver (r = .433, p = .008). Finally, the results showed there was no statistically significant relationship between the weekly hours a caregiver spent providing care and subjective wellbeing (r = .119, p = .489).

The results of the correlation analysis in Table 5 show there was a statistically significant relationship between the self-efficacy of the research participants and subjective wellbeing (r = . 352, p = .035), providing support for Hypothesis 1 indicating there would be a positive relationship between self-efficacy and subjective wellbeing. The results also showed there was a statistically significant relationship between the social support of the research

Table 4.Correlation Analysis: Control Variables on Subjective Wellbeing

Variable	*r*	*P*
Age	.118	.492
Gender	.043	.804
Gross Income	.192	.262
Months	.433	.008**
Hours	.119	.489

Note. p <. 05* p < .01**

participants and subjective wellbeing ($r = .385, p = .020$), providing support for Hypothesis 2 indicating there would be a positive relationship between social support and subjective wellbeing. Next, the results showed there was no statistically significant relationship between the resilience of the research participants and subjective wellbeing ($r = .175, p = .309$), running counter to Hypothesis 3 indicating there would be a positive relationship between resilience and subjective wellbeing. The results also showed there was a statistically significant relationship between the spirituality of the research participants and subjective wellbeing ($r = .342, p = .041$), providing support for Hypothesis 4 indicating there would be a positive relationship between spirituality and subjective wellbeing. The results further showed there was a statistically significant relationship between the leisure participation of the research participants and subjective wellbeing ($r = .353, p = .035$), providing support for Hypothesis 5 indicating there would be a positive relationship between leisure participation and subjective wellbeing.

Table 6 shows the results of the stepwise regression analysis. In the equation in Table 6, the number of months caregivers spent providing care to the care recipients was the only significant predictor ($b = .009, p = .008$) of the subjective wellbeing of informal caregivers. Other variables, such as gender, age, gross income, the weekly hours that caregivers spent providing care, self-efficacy, social support, resilience, spirituality, and leisure participation, dropped out of the analysis as significant predictors of subjective wellbeing. The adjusted R-square for the model was .163.

Analysis of Qualitative Data

This section presents the results from the qualitative segment of the instrument used in this study. Creswell (2009) suggested that researchers can analyze qualitative data using the following categories:

Table 5.Correlation Analysis: Independent Variables on Subjective Wellbeing

Variable	r	p
Self-Efficacy	.352	.035*
Social Support	.385	.020*
Resilience	.175	.309
Spirituality	.342	.041*
Leisure Participation	.353	.035*

Note. $p <. 05^*$ $p < .01^{**}$

Table 6.Regression Equation Predicting Subjective Wellbeing (Results of Stepwise Regression; N = 36)

Variable	Coefficient	Standard Error	*p*
Intercept	6.797	.273	.000
Months	.009	.003	.008

R-Square = .187
Adj. R. Square = .163
F statistic = 7.824
Sig F = .008
p <..05* p <.01**

- Codes on topics that readers would expect to find based on past literature and common sense.
- Codes that are surprising and not anticipated at the beginning of the study.
- Codes that are unusual and that are, in and of themselves, of conceptual interest to readers.
- Codes that address a larger theoretical perspective in the research.

Table 7 contains quotes that readers will expect to find based on past literature and common sense as suggested by Creswell (2009). The table presents participants' anticipated responses (n = 21) regarding how their caregiving responsibilities affected their subjective wellbeing.

On the basis of the information provided above, the researcher formulated the following proposition, which is also a reflection of the result of the hypothesis testing presented regarding the nature of subjective wellbeing. The qualitative results showed that most of the research participants (n = 19) believed their caregiving responsibilities adversely affected their subjective wellbeing.

Table 8 presents participants' unanticipated responses (n = 8) regarding how their caregiving responsibilities affected their subjective wellbeing.

On the basis of the information provided above, the researcher formulated the following proposition, which is also a reflection of the result of the hypothesis testing presented regarding the nature of subjective wellbeing. Some of the research participants (n = 8) believed their caregiving responsibilities had a positive psychological effect on their subjective wellbeing.

Table 9 presents participants' unusual responses (n = 3) regarding how their caregiving responsibilities affected their subjective wellbeing.

Table 7.Anticipated Responses (Subjective Wellbeing)

Case No.	Anticipated (Subjective Wellbeing)
1	Being a caregiver affects my ability to maintain the quality of life I desire because it is a strain on my mental capacity and physical appearance. I cannot focus at school sometimes and don't have time to appear as presentable as I please.
2	Caregiving is often emotionally and physically exhausting. Working a full-time job and caring for a loved one at home can be very overwhelming. Limited access to travel or enjoy relaxing downtime. Everything revolves around the person being cared for.
3	Not able to be spontaneous affects my quality of life, for example wanting to travel on a whim is not possible because of my caregiving duties. Basic things like meal planning, transportation, medical appointments, entertaining company has to be arranged. The stress of dealing with these issues and others that are the caregiver's responsibility can have a negative effect on your quality of life. Especially if you have to tackle it alone. You must be resourceful to handle it.
6	As a caregiver you usually must provide 100% quality care which often leaves you with much less time for providing or doing things for yourself. This affects your quality of life.
7	It's difficult but I am committed to taking care of family. This is not something I ever imagined; however, I stand-up to the challenge.
8	Because using monies earned to pay for incontinence products makes me not able to afford things I could before. So that affects my quality of life.
10	Providing care for my grandfather significantly limits the time I have to take care of my household tasks or spend time with my friends.
13	Being a single mother and caregiver for my aging parent affects my personal time, my ability to socialize with friends, physical upkeep, and my romantic relationships.
15	My quality of life is affected because normally I'd spend much of my time with friends, taking trips, shopping, movies, etc. Because my parent is here, I'm aware that they can't be left alone [and] this prevents me from traveling, etc. Plus I feel guilty if I leave her.
16	I am not as active as I would like since caregiving for my husband began. So that affects my happiness sometimes and I feel down. Then I think of earlier years and how things were and I come around.
18	It impacts the time that I have to do personal things that I choose to put on the back burner so I can be available.
21	It is virtually impossible to travel or leave for extended periods of time. You must always be "on call," concerned that there might be an emergency at home. So my quality of life has changed drastically since I became a caregiver. I am more stressed.
22	Overall responsibility of someone is very hard on a daily basis. So it's very hard to be focused on yourself or anything else other than the person you are caring for.
23	Providing care for my parent at times does not allow me to do certain things that I desire such as yoga, working overtime, gardening, etc.
26	My role as a caregiver affects my ability to maintain the quality of life I am accustomed to. Things have changed. I have to make several personal sacrifices to care for my mom.
29	The act of caregiving leaves little time or energy or resources for any other activities that bring pleasure or additional finances.
30	My role as a caregiver affects my ability to maintain the quality of life I desire because I'm always tired from caregiving duties. It's rare that I have the energy to do anything other than caring from my mom.
31	Being a caregiver to my mom affects my ability to maintain the quality of life I desire because caring for her demands about 80% of my time. Seeing to her daily care, my job, her doctor, it's really trying but I thank God she is here for me to take care of her. I have no complaints lord!
34	The only thing that it takes from me is time.

Table 8. Unanticipated Responses (Subjective Wellbeing)

Case No.	Unanticipated (Subjective Wellbeing)
4	Helping others as a caregiver gives a wonderful sense of accomplishment and satisfaction knowing that you're helping others at a time when they need it most.
17	I devote time caring for my loved ones (mother and stepmother, and father). Even so I am still able to work some time so not that much.
25	My quality of life remains the same as a caregiver. I know mom is aging and my child can be sickly. But my situation is better than others I know.
27	Being a caregiver is such an honor. It gives me great joy. This is what keeps me going. This is what I have been called to do.
28	As a caregiver of a relative that is young it can get to be hard to see them with the illness, but you love them so much it gives you that drive, that quality of life to keep going because you know it's the right thing to do.
32	It makes me feel blessed to be able to take care of my dad, before my dad I took care of my mother. I believe this is what God intended me to do.
33	I should've had my personal issues in check long before my mom's stroke. Now being able to finally sit still for a couple of hours during the day that I spend with her has allowed me to start clearing my mind and seeing things better. The only thing I can't do is have enough time to get my household chores done because of being with mom and taking her to therapy 3 days a week.
36	I try to ensure that I keep my life as normal as possible before I assumed this role as a caregiver. I don't mean to appear selfish but I must be sure my life remains somewhat the same in terms of the things I did and all that. I must stay encouraged unless everything falters.

Table 9.Unusual (Subjective Wellbeing)

Case No.	Unusual (Subjective Wellbeing)
9	It gives me an ideal on how to live my life. How to make quality decisions on the foods I eat, how important exercise is, and to remember to make time for recreation with family and friends.
12	Sitting down and thinking it out before I made my move to take care of my mom. Knowing the ins and outs of other people I had seen being cared for I put my plan into action.
14	Being a caregiver has no effect on my quality of life.

The participants provided no responses that addressed larger theoretical perspectives.

Table 10 addresses codes related to participants' perceptions of self-efficacy.

On the basis of the information provided above, the researcher formulated the following proposition, which is also a reflection of the result of the hypothesis testing presented regarding the nature of self-efficacy. The qualitative results showed that a significant number of research participants (n = 17) believed they were innately capable of handling their caregiving responsibilities.

Table 10.Anticipated (Self Efficacy)

Case No.	Anticipated (Self-Efficacy)
1	I am a leader and I'm quick on my feet so most problems in my environment don't faze me. I can take on any task.
2	As a working full-time employee with taxing responsibilities the duties associated with caring for a dependent parent often seem daunting. Yet the experience has made me very capable in multitasking.
3	Being able to solve problems quickly and efficiently makes me feel as though I can take on the challenge of caring for someone other than myself even if their health is not always the best.
4	As a caregiver, I am in charge of a person's wellbeing, so I take it seriously and try to be proactive in stimulating them in the ways that I can, at the same time allowing them the right of independence and the satisfaction that comes with it.
6	If you are gifted to be a caregiver, it will show in various ways; mostly positive. Therefore the impact in the role of a caregiver is exhibited in your actions.
7	I worked in the medical field working with patients for ten years. I learned how to do a lot of the treatments and procedures I use now when caring for my aunt. I know the experience then helps me tremendously now in my present situation.
9	My belief that I could handle this task comforts me in my role as a caregiver.
11	I strongly believe my capabilities as a caregiver helps me perform the tasks required of me. Actually I find it easy to do what's required.
14	I believe that I am very capable of my responsibilities in my role as a caregiver.
16	Yes, I am strongly confident in my belief that I am extremely capable of the requirements that I must handle as a caregiver. So I can handle things. But I do appreciate a little help now and then.
21	You must believe that the overriding priority is the best interest of your parent. I recognize the limitations of my capabilities and seek home health professionals to help me.
22	Mainly because I love the person I am caring for and when you love people it help you handle the biggest responsibility of caregiving.
23	I know I am capable and able to perform my task in the role. I believe when you are confident you perform well.
26	Because I am a responsible person I know how to multi-task and reach my objective as a caregiver.
27	I believe I am capable of learning more and solving problems after thinking about the situation.
30	My capabilities as a caregiver impact my responsibilities in that role because I know exactly what to do in any given situation. My cousin is a certified nursing assistant and has helped me by teaching me the proper steps to help my mom. If she unexpectedly has a seizure, I know the proper steps to keep that her safe.
31	I believe because I am a caregiver to my mom my capabilities are endless. I will do all I can for her no matter what it takes. There is nothing to hard or to difficult when it comes to her care. An example is when her prescription for her blood thinning meds was held up. I moved mountains and actually reached her doctor on a Sunday morning to get her medications started. Thank you Jesus!

Table 11 presents participants' unanticipated responses ($n = 14$) regarding how their caregiving responsibilities affected their self-efficacy.

On the basis of the information provided above, the researcher formulated the following proposition derived from unanticipated responses, which is also a reflection of the result of the hypothesis testing presented regarding the nature of self-efficacy. An ample number of research participants ($n = 14$) relied on their religious convictions as the lynchpin to sustaining their self-efficacy levels in their roles as informal caregivers as it related to their subjective wellbeing. The participants provided no responses that were unusual or addressed larger theoretical perspectives.

Tables 12 and 13 address codes related to participants' perceptions of social support.

Table 11. Unanticipated (Self-Efficacy)

Case No.	Unanticipated (Self-Efficacy)
5	My personal beliefs teach me to love and care for all especially family.
8	When family gets involved sometimes they make bad decisions. I had to intervene to make sure the decisions were normal and in the best interest of my grandparents.
10	I don't believe I have enough experience or insight to provide care for an older family member due to my age.
12	Thinking it out long before I made the responsibility to take care of mommy.
13	My role as a caregiver requires me to be solution focused at all times.
15	I've found most problems have a solution. The difficulty is getting CLEAR information about an issue, to arrive at a rational solution. With an elderly parent, I have to decide if she has a real physical ailment or if she's just upset and simply seeking attention.
17	I strongly believe and know that God is doing this thru me; there is no other way. During trying days I would encourage myself by saying, "Is not going to always be like this." It will get better and guess what it does get better. I am determined that every day is a good day.
20	Trust in the Lord with all your heart and lean not on your own understandings. In all your ways acknowledge him and he shall direct your paths (Proverbs 3: 5-6).
25	The fact that I love the individual and my religious foundation motivates my care.
29	I believe I am resilient and resourceful. As a caregiver, I roll with the punches, deal with the unexpected, and try to fortify myself to deal with future challenges.
32	I worked in the medical field for years before taking on caregiving to my dad I took care of others.
33	Honestly, this is something Blacks have done from generation to generation. I learned from a young child that faith would take you a long way. Life will throw many obstacles in your way. Being able to multi-task is a must in my family.
34	I'm a caring God-fearing person and God can solve all problems.
36	I am usually a very patient person who does not lose insight on who is the patient and our roles do not become reverse.

Table 12. Anticipated (Social Support)

Case No.	Anticipated (Social Support)
1	I believe that social support, my personality, and personal experiences do impact my role as a caregiver. When my friends say encouraging words or I overhear the experiences from other family members, I know that things will be okay. It is good to have people around you; then you are better with them.
2	Often my friends know when I need some time for relaxation and they are persistent in encouraging me to take time for myself. I realize that I am not superwoman and cannot do everything without help. Luckily whenever I ask, support is available. That's important for me.
3	Sharing my feelings with others is a respite and reinvigorates me.
4	My friends and family allow me to "vent" basically express myself, state my concerns, and reveal my challenges. They also give me constructive ways to handle situations that arise. They are a great support to me and very encouraging so I am more prepared.
5	I appreciate when people come over to visit and talk just to empower me. It helps me.
6	The more support you have, the better caregiver you can be.
7	A dear friend has been a real help in directing me to handle major issues like getting social services and navigating the medical system. She has directed me to various resources to assist in caring for my elderly aunt. I know her support has been invaluable.
8	My friends help me a lot. I could call then at times and just talk or even cry. This is good for me and makes me a better caregiver.
9	The support of others helps me emotionally during this experience, then you can continue on.
10	Support from family can make or break you. Unfortunately, family typically has to rearrange their schedules to allow you as the caregiver to receive time away from your family member that is in need of care. Without a large group of support, it would be impossible to provide care and maintain a good quality of life.
11	I get information from others in similar situations. This gives me the support I need. I can talk with someone just like me to get advice.
12	I have people who were going through this long before me. I saw this thing and I knew I was going to take on my part in the role to be played. It helps me that folks had been there, too.
13	Support from friends and family helps me be open-minded and secure about choices I make as a caregiver.
14	Yes it allows me to take care of myself.
16	Support from my family and friends make it easier for me to provide the care required by Mr. [Name]. I would be really stressed without their support.
18	It helps me take some of the pressure off.
21	It is imperative that the caregiver has a life outside of caring for the patient. When you have that support you are able to provide more intense and a better quality of caregiving service.
22	Other people give you another way of looking at a situation. This can impact your caregiving in a positive way.
23	Since I have a great support system, obstacles don't seem so large and overwhelming. Being able to openly and honestly talk things out with someone makes the stress easier.
25	The testimony of their life experience and shared values gives me a ballast to handle things.
26	Support from other people allow me to talk about whatever is going on in my life as a sounding board which continue to allow me to care for my mom effectively.
27	Support from others allowed me to participate in other interest.

Case No.	Anticipated (Social Support)
29	It is nice to know that I have a support system that I can go to for comfort and to vet ideas. That is the way in which family and friends are there for me. They cannot be more than that and I don't expect them to. They have their own challenging lives and problems.
30	The support from other people helps me to keep pushing. Being a caregiver is not easy and it's good to have people around you that are rooting for your success.
32	I get the praise from family for taking on the responsibility but I would do it anyway.
33	My sisters and I are our own support system. My mom took excellent care of us and we're in this 100% taking care of her.
34	Some people may have experience in the caregiving role and their experience helps me to be a better caregiver in certain situations.
36	They help me to release my tension by listening to my concerns. Having someone to share my feelings help me to understand my role as a caregiver.

On the basis of the information provided above, the researcher formulated the following proposition, which is also a reflection of the result of the hypothesis testing presented regarding the nature of social support. A substantial number of research participants ($n = 28$) perceived that a socially supportive environment encompassing family, friends, and the surrounding community was an essential ingredient in enhancing their ability to perform their caregiver responsibilities and maintaining their subjective wellbeing.

In responding to the open-ended questions regarding social support, there were no discernible patterns or themes pertaining to the codes that were categorized as unanticipated, unusual, or those addressing larger theoretical perspectives.

Tables 13 and 14 address codes related to participants' perceptions of spirituality.

On the basis of the information provided above, the researcher formulated the following proposition, which is also a reflection of the result of the hypothesis testing presented regarding the nature of spirituality. The vast majority of the research participants ($n = 32$) had the perception that their spiritual beliefs were positively influential to their caregiving roles and their subjective wellbeing.

In responding to the open-ended questions pertaining to spirituality, there were no significantly discernible themes pertaining to the codes that were categorized as unanticipated, unusual, or those addressing larger theoretical perspectives. The only exception was one case in which there was an unusual code indicating a detached connection to the belief in God.

Table 13 Anticipated (Spirituality)

Case No.	**Anticipated (Spirituality)**
1	Spirituality affects my beliefs and that impacts my role as a caregiver. It guides my daily decisions and lightens my heart.
2	My spirituality affects my role as a caregiver through the strong faith in God it provides me. I believe it is God who is carrying me daily through this difficult situation. My spirituality sustains me even when I feel like giving up.
3	I believe and feel that God will not give me more than I can bear. So understanding that gives me the tenacity I need to handle the challenges I face.
4	My spirituality and faith in God and his word the Bible guide and direct me in my role as a caregiver. It is the force behind what I do for others and how I treat those in my care. Spirituality teaches me to be a kind, considerate, and compassionate caregiver.
5	I am to love and care for all those that I care for and love.
6	As a caregiver, spirituality is so important. It is definitely what gets you through the day.
7	My belief is strong enough to keep me motivated to know that God has my back all the way through times like this. The life lessons I have also enable me to withstand these types of situations.
8	With Christ I am able to make decisions based in Christian faith for my grandparents.
9	My spirituality makes me understand that a personal relationship with God is very important. It also helps me know how important it is to take care of the elderly.
10	My spirituality allows me to remain focused on his care. I believe that if I didn't rely on my spirituality, I honestly would've neglected his care more. Spirituality is a huge motivation for doing the right thing.
11	I was raised to be kind to people, which affects my spiritual connection to others.
12	My life was on the line each day in my job because I worked for 15 years as a lineman for [Company]. So spirituality is always in my heart. It helps everything that I do.
13	My spirituality helps me stay balanced in my emotions.
14	My spirituality makes me able to adapt to any problem in my caregiver role. I am always prayed up.
16	My spirituality affects my caregiver role because I made a vow before God that I would support this man in sickness and in health. If I broke that vow my spirit would feel bad.
17	My relationship with Almighty God is the key. I don't see this as work. I see this as ministry. Everywhere I go I'm trying to find someone that I can be a blessing to and especially to my child.
18	I look and seek God. He directs my path and gives me patience in stressful situations. So yes, being a spiritual being makes me a more conscience caregiver.
21	When caregiving for someone with a terminal illness you know there will be an end. Spirituality makes the end bearable because you know that God will take the reins when its time.
22	Spirituality makes me love my spouse harder and be more patient.
23	I always use my faith and prayer on a daily basis to make it through hard times and praise God for the good times.
25	My spirituality gives me strength to deal with the person I'm caring for and the ups and downs of caregiving.
26	My spirituality affects my role as a caregiver 100%. I do everything based on the love of God. God served his people and because I'm living to be Christ-like. I must follow his way.

Case No.	Anticipated (Spirituality)
27	Spirituality affects my role as a caregiver because I feel all things in life are lessons God teaches us. As a caregiver I learn more each time.
28	God tells us to love one another in Luke 4 you will find that Satan tempted Jesus, hoping to find an area of weakness. Jesus stood strong and defeated the enemy. So we have to stand strong pray and know God can, and HE will fulfill all of our needs.
29	My spirituality is what renews and reinvigorates me. It also keeps me grounded and reminds me of something bigger than myself operating. I like to think it (in the form of instinct and intuition) guides me in my decision-making and my treatment of others.
30	My spiritual beliefs affect everything I do in life. As a caregiver, my spirituality keeps me leveled.
31	If I didn't have Jesus I don't know where I would be. I am so thankful for the holy spirit being in me. If I were left to think or act on my own, Lord, I don't want to think about the kind of person I would be. The serene peace I receive when I am going thru especially in times such as this, when I talk to my Lord and Savior. He gives me guidance and serene peace in the midst of storms and he helps me see my way thru. This is how I am able to put one foot in front of the other every day and I am able to think and care for my mom! I thank you Lord! Hallelujah! Thank you Jesus!
32	Through God all things are possible. Whenever I don't know the answer I pray about it. If I think that Dad is not feeling well and won't tell me I just wait for a sign.
33	Every living thing or being shall die and in between if you don't turn your life over to Christ and receive the Holy Spirit; Pray, have faith, you need that relationship; without it you're dead.
34	No one's perfect. I pray and I ask the Lord for help mostly every day. This relationship impacts my role as a caregiver it guides my decisions and comforts my spirit.
35	It is a must!
36	It keeps me praying and it seems to guide me with decisions I have to make regarding this person's care. The spirit guides me by letting me know exactly when she is feeling low and then doing just the right thing to perk her up.

Tables 14 and 15 address codes related to participants' perceptions of leisure participation.

On the basis of the information provided above, the researcher formulated the following proposition, which is also a reflection of the result of the hypothesis testing presented regarding the nature of leisure participation. Most of the research participants (n = 21) believed their involvement in leisure activities was critical to their role as informal caregivers and vital for their subjective wellbeing.

A significant number of the research participants (n = 10) believed they had limited time for leisure activities, but this did not negatively affect their performance as informal caregivers. A careful inspection of the interview data showed there were no unusual codes or issues related to the formulation of larger theoretical propositions.

Table 14 Anticipated (Leisure Participation)

Case No.	Anticipated (Leisure Participation)
1	Leisure activities like going to a concert, taking a short trip, or just hanging out does give me that extra push. Participation in these activities makes me return to caregiving fresh and ready to perform.
3	Having activities and interests outside the home is like a retreat! Outside leisure activities nourish my soul and invigorates me. This allows me to push ahead.
4	I try to take time and schedule time for leisure activities. I realize the leisure activities play a role in my wellbeing to give me joy and enjoyment, and to refresh me and reinvigorate me to continue as a whole person, a better caregiver.
6	As a caregiver your leisure time is quite limited. However, the more leisure you can do would make your situation somewhat more manageable.
8	Leisure participation helps a lot to release steam and it gives time to have fun.
9	Leisure activities are great for a caregiver. It provides relief for the caregiver.
11	I stay active in leisure things like exercising, reading, and football. This helps me release any stress I might have and remain calm in my role.
12	It is important to let off the steam one builds up inside. Over time, sister and I understand "you weekends and I got her Monday – Friday." That way we both got a little time for fun stuff. It's important for you.
13	Leisure activities are important to keeping a balance in your life. I strive to create time for leisure activities as well as maintaining the support needed for my caregiver role.
16	My participation in sports (golf and bowling) affects me positively because it provides an outlet for the tension that caregiving causes.
17	I see things totally different. This is my leisure. I don't know if you understand, but for me this is fun. There is so much joy in being a caregiver. I LOVE IT!
21	My participation in leisure activities rejuvenates me and allows me to take a breath from what can be an emotionally draining journey. I am then in a more relaxed state for the difficult times ahead.
25	Fellowshipping is important. Gathering with people you love is very important. It feeds the spirit. Everyone needs to belong to a group for support.
26	Participating with activities helps me to be a better caregiver because having some "me time" allows me to become more energized and continue to care for my mom.
27	I am able to spend time with family and friends due to shared time.
28	My leisure activities are church fellowshipping with church family, and friends, maybe a dinner out with friends.
29	It is very important that I take time for pleasurable leisure activities with loved ones. If I do not give myself that gift, I am a lot less able to be my "best self." This shows up in my decision-making, interpersonal interactions, and quality of care I provide.
30	Participating in leisure activities keeps me up to date, up to beat, and happier than ever.
32	We have a lot of family functions, I do all the cooking because my house is the family house and I don't have to take dad out. I cook a lot of food it gives me peace and joy. We have a large family and they look forward to eating my cooking and that pleases me.
33	I was a workaholic. I really never had time for leisure time. So last year God allowed me to work part-time from full-time hours and me and my mom are starting to get out more. She was always taking care of someone else. Never taking time for herself after her retirement. So now God has given us a second chance and it's all about my mom so I make sure that every 3 months we get out of here and do something leisurely.
34	My leisure activities are caring for my grandkids, family, and friends. I love God, my family, and my church family.
32	We have a lot of family functions, I do all the cooking because my house is the family house and I don't have to take dad out. I cook a lot of food it gives me peace and joy. We have a large family and they look forward to eating my cooking and that pleases me.

Table 15 Unanticipated (Leisure Participation)

Case No.	Unanticipated (Leisure Participation)
2	My limited resources and the fact that my mom's limitations require that someone be with her constantly does not allow me to participate in a lot of leisure.
5	Unfortunately, in my case since my stepmom now lives with me there is very little time for leisure. I believe that it would help though.
7	I have very little if any time for myself. I sometimes forget to eat. My spare time is spent catching up on household stuff. That's it.
10	Being a caregiver requires me to forego spending time with my family and friends.
14	None because I have other members to help.
15	I am going to attempt to get my parent into a senior citizens' activity group of some kind. If I can accomplish that, I can re-inflate my social life.
18	I would like to have more leisure time but circumstances put me in a place where I need to make choices and right now the choice is my mom. I asked God to keep her and I want to do my part willingly.
22	Usually if I have downtime I spend it doing some cleaning or other household stuff. My leisure time is different now I use it to catch up on stuff.
31	Being a caregiver to my mom I have no time for leisure activities. If I were able to get someone that she is comfortable with to sit with her, maybe then there would be a possibility that I could have some leisure time, when I do have time is when I just get her together and take her with me. She needs to have pampered days more than me. She really enjoys getting manicures and pedicures. I enjoy seeing her smile and feel good with all she has been through. So again I give God all the glory for all that he is doing in her recovery. I give him all the praise in Jesus name, Amen!!!!
36	Being a caregiver limits my outside activities because I am constantly thinking I need to do something for her to ensure she is comfortable and enjoying herself.

Tables 16 and 17 address codes related to participants' perceptions of resilience.

On the basis of the information provided above, the researcher formulated the following proposition, which is also a reflection of the result of the hypothesis testing presented regarding the nature of resilience. The vast majority of research participants ($n = 20$) believed resilience allowed them to be optimistic about their performance as caregivers.

On the basis of the information provided above, the researcher formulated the following proposition, which also is a reflection of the result of the hypothesis testing presented regarding the nature of resilience. Several of the research participants ($n = 10$) expressed myriad unanticipated responses that did not address the central issue of whether resilience affected their role as a caregiver. Yet, they did address how their spiritual beliefs provided them the resolve necessary in handling their caregiver responsibilities. There were no unusual codes identified in the data or codes that reflected larger theoretical perspectives.

Table 16 Anticipated (Resilience)

Case No.	Anticipated (Resilience)
1	My resilience helps me not to panic. It gives me the strength to believe that I can handle this situation. I am able to easily piece situations that seem chaotic back together again.
3	I can always see the bright side of a less than optimal situation. Therefore, my optimism helps me to be positive about future outcomes.
4	I try to face each day anew and not allow past events or challenges to affect how I treat my spouse even when I'm feeling stressed I don't let it influence how I handle myself during his care. It takes a lot of resilience to maintain your composure.
5	My resilience just helps me have patience and try to understand we all may need help in one way or another at some time during our life.
9	My level of resilience greatly affects my role as a caregiver because it makes me move ahead no matter what occurs.
11	I believe that my past experience and jobs have helped me a lot.
13	My level of resilience helps me deal with the needs of my parents because I must keep up my stamina to give good care.
14	My resilience is very strong as a caregiver. That helps me stay strong and ready for whatever.
15	Gather information, focus on the given problem, solve it, and move on.
16	Generally I am able to recover when the day has been challenging. I believe that tomorrow may be better but even if not I will continue to move forward because it is my duty to do so.
18	It actually strengthens me and helps me to look at the situation objectively.
21	Resilience is imperative. Caregiving is a marathon, not a sprint. There is a beginning seemingly with no end in sight. Your ability to bounce back from the tougher days will be your best resolve for this challenge.
22	I am not a quitter I continue to push forward until I make it through.
23	No matter what happens or why it happens it never stops me from reaching goals or providing care for my parents.
25	I think my level of resilience affects my caregiving skills because I can separate my experiences, not take things personally, and then continue to treat her.
26	My level of resilience does not affect my role as a caregiver in a negative way. I like to look ahead to problem solve situations that may occur.
27	My level of resilience depends on the activity. If our activities include things she enjoys and she's happy, then I am ok. If her challenges are more trying, it's more difficult because I want to find ways to help her.
29	My resilience helps me tremendously. Both in my own ability to keep going when under tremendous stress and in my ability to encourage/support/motivate the person I am caring for . . . and other family and friends when needed.
34	My resilience allows me to be able to tackle any situation at any given time.
36	As a caregiver sometimes I reflect on the past to build up my strength because it helps me to continue my role as a caretaker; knowing what this person has done for me during my childhood years.

Table 17. Unanticipated (Resilience)

Case No.	Unanticipated (Resilience)
2	My willpower has been significantly strained since the death of my younger sibling. This has also influenced the decline of my parent's health, too.
6	I wish I were more resilient when setbacks occur in my life but I am working on it. If I were more resilient I would not fall down as a caregiver.
7	I have a strong belief in God, which has increased and given me the strength I need now. My strength has always helped me in tough situations in my life. That's how I just keep right on trucking.
8	I was to go through the motions of when the parents are forgetting to help my grandparents. Then I have to be there to make the decisions for them. This makes me strong enough to know I can care for them too.
10	It's difficult to maintain focus of my long-term goals while maintaining care for my grandfather.
12	My grandmother has 10 children and I have always played the role as her gofer so I was all over the households.
30	Since nothing really keeps me down I try to stay happy when taking care of my mom. I never really let what is happening affect my care for my mom.
31	There are blows that I have taken in life that have knocked me down and I took my time to get up. But seeing my mom down and out from the stroke, I don't let anything keep me down or stop me from being there for her. I take a minute to pause and gather myself then it's back to business. I know prayer does change things. Thank you Jesus!
32	I pray about everything and take it one day at a time.
33	I thank God that I haven't experienced anything that was too hard to come through. But with God we know all things are possible. It helps when you have strong faith and a praying family. I've had some really bad days. I didn't know how or what was going to happen, but I keep thanking God anyway.

The researcher discovered during the analysis of the qualitative responses to the open-ended queries that the participants' replies provided some support for each of the hypotheses. In particular, there were very constructive responses for the variables of leisure participation, social support, and spirituality with regard to the significance of these constructs on subjective wellbeing. These views aligned closely with the participants' quantitative responses to the survey.

CONCLUSION

This chapter presented a restatement of the research purpose, descriptive statistics for the continuous and categorical variables, and results of the hypothesis testing. There were five null hypotheses formulated to address the research question. Pearson correlations and regression analyses were performed to address all the stipulated null hypotheses.

The results of the correlation analysis showed there was a statistically significant relationship between the subjective wellbeing of the research participants and the following independent variables: self-efficacy, social support, leisure participation, and spirituality. There was no statistically significant relationship between the subjective wellbeing and the resilience of the research participants.

A stepwise regression analysis was also performed. The results showed the number of months caregivers spent providing care to the care recipients was the only significant predictor of the subjective wellbeing of the informal caregivers who participated in this study. Other variables, such as gender, age, gross income, weekly hours informal caregivers provided care, self-efficacy, social support, resilience, and spirituality, were not significant predictors of subjective wellbeing in this particular analysis. This result was likely related to the small sample size and did not provide much additional insight regarding the hypothesized relationships.

This researcher developed several generalizations about the variables that affect the subjective wellbeing of informal caregivers in terms of emerging patterns and themes and how they compared and contrasted with the extant literature on the subject being investigated (Creswell, 2009). Some of these patterns, in varying degrees, were also consistent with the results of the above inferential statistical analyses. This method of correlating responses was somewhat reinforced in Onwuegbuzie and Teddie (2003). Hence, the researchers formulated the following propositions and themes on the basis of the open-ended responses to questions attached to the survey instrument:

- Most of the research participants believed their caregiving responsibilities adversely affected their subjective wellbeing.
- Some of the research participants believed their caregiving responsibilities had a positive psychological effect on their subjective wellbeing.
- A significant number of research participants believed they were innately capable of handling their caregiving responsibilities.
- Research participants had the perception that their spiritual beliefs were positively influential to their caregiver roles and their subjective wellbeing.
- Research participants relied on their spiritual convictions as the lynchpin in sustaining themselves in their roles as informal caregivers as it related to their subjective wellbeing.

- Research participants perceived that a socially supportive environment encompassing family, friends, and the surrounding community was an essential ingredient in enhancing their ability to perform their caregiver responsibilities and maintaining their subjective wellbeing.
- The vast majority of research participants believed their resilience allowed them to be optimistic about their performance as caregivers.
- Most of the research participants believed their participation in leisure activities was critical to their role as informal caregivers and vital for their subjective wellbeing.
- A significant number of the research participants believed they had limited time for leisure activities but felt this did not negatively affect their performance as informal caregivers.

REFERENCES

Green, S. N., & Salkind, N. J. (2016). *Using SPSS for Windows and Macintosh*. London: Pearson.

Onwuegbuzie, A. J., & Teddie, C. (2003). A framework for analyzing data in mixed methods research. In A. Tashakkori & C. Teddie (Eds.), *Handbook of mixed methods in social and behavioral sciences*. Thousand Oaks, CA: Sage Publications.

Pallent, J. (2013). *A step by step guide to data analysis using IBM SPSS*. London: Open University Press.

Verma, J. P. (2013). *Data analysis in management with SPSS Software*. New Delhi: Springer. doi:10.1007/978-81-322-0786-3

ADDITIONAL READING

Burhan, K. P., & Johnson, D. H. (2001). Suggestions for presenting results of data analysis. *The Journal of Wildlife Management*, *65*(3), 373–378. doi:10.2307/3803088

Ellis, P. D. (2010). *The essential guide to effect sizes: Statistical power, meta-analysis, and the interpretation of research results*. Cambridge, UK: Cambridge University Press. doi:10.1017/CBO9780511761676

Lewis, S. (2015). Qualitative inquiry and research design: Choosing among five approaches. *Health Promotion Practice*, *16*(4), 473–475. doi:10.1177/1524839915580941

Chapter 4
Discussion and Policy Recommendations

ABSTRACT

This chapter encapsulates discussion of research findings and their relevant policy conclusions and recommendations. Thus, it is suggested that there was no statistically significant relationship between the age of respondents and their subjective wellbeing. This finding contradicts the results of an early study conducted by Fluegel. Results of the current study also revealed there was no statistically significant relationship between gender and the subjective wellbeing of respondents. Similarly, the results also demonstrate there was no statistically significant relationship between gross income and the subjective wellbeing of respondents. It is suggested that these results coincide with a study conducted by Gaynor. Results of the other independent variables are also discussed in this chapter. These include self-efficacy, social support, resilience, spirituality, and leisure participation. These results are compared and contrasted from the qualitative results in identifying meaningful patterns, similarities, and variances.

INTRODUCTION

This chapter contains a discussion of the research findings presented in the previous chapter. References are also made to the stated research question and hypotheses. Further, the categories used to analyze the qualitative segment of the survey instrument are presented along with the results of

DOI: 10.4018/978-1-5225-7452-1.ch004

testing the five stipulated null hypotheses. In addition, the chapter contains a delineation of the essential research objective as well as a report on the results of hypotheses testing. This chapter also examines the meaning of the results of hypotheses testing within a broader context of the extant literature. Conclusions and suggestions are rendered regarding future directions in empirical and theoretical research on itinerant overt and latent variables that affect the subjective wellbeing or mental health of informal caregivers as well as policy development.

RESTATEMENT OF THE RESEARCH OBJECTIVE

Invariably, this study had one primary and particular objective. This objective embodies the implementation of a mixed methods concurrent research design geared at examining the factors that influence the subjective wellbeing of informal caregivers. These factors include self-efficacy, spirituality, social support, resilience, and leisure participation. The major gap in the research literature this study was designed to address was the paucity of empirical studies regarding issues of emotional episodes, financial stress, ill health, and an increased risk of mortality experienced by informal caregivers (Cohen et al., 2002; Haley et al., 2003; Robinson, 1983). To address the research question, the researchers developed testable statistical hypotheses. These null hypotheses were used to examine the relationships between subjective wellbeing and the predictor variables so defined in previous chapters.

In addition, the researcher analyzed the qualitative segment of the instrument using the following categories as suggested by Creswell (2007):

- Codes on topics that readers would expect to find based on the past literature and common sense.
- Codes that are surprising and were not anticipated at the beginning of the study.
- Codes that are unusual and that are, in and of themselves, of conceptual interest to readers.
- Codes that address a larger theoretical perspective in the research.

Results of Hypotheses Testing

Results of this study indicated there was no statistically significant relationship between the age of respondents and their subjective wellbeing, which contradicted the results of an early study conducted by Fluegel (1925, pp. 345-346). Fluegel assessed the moods of nine respondents (five females and four males) by asking them to diary their emotional events. However, he did not gauge the effect of chronological age on subjects' subjective wellbeing. Another notable difference between Fluegel's work and the current study was the different indices used to measure subjective wellbeing. However, other studies were an improvement on the study conducted by Fluegel. For example, after 1945, researchers began using short and simple questionnaires to ask individuals about their happiness levels and life satisfaction. A clear example of this change was the 1969 study carried out by Bradburn.

Additionally, results of the current study revealed there was no statistically significant relationship between gender and the subjective wellbeing of respondents. Also, there was no statistically significant relationship between gross income and the subjective wellbeing of respondents.

The results indicated there was a statistically significant relationship between the number of months caregivers spent providing care to the recipients and their subjective wellbeing. These results coincide with the Gaynor (1988) study mentioned earlier, which indicated that caregivers offering care for longer periods of time expressed increased burden compared to caregivers with shorter caregiving experiences. Yet, results of the current study reflected there was no statistically significant relationship between the weekly hours a caregiver spent providing care and subjective wellbeing.

These findings confirmed research conducted by Diener (2000) on subjective wellbeing. However, readers should note that findings of an earlier work by Diener and Diener (1996) are counterintuitive when placed in the broader context of the findings presented in the current study. Thus, this is so because Diener tended to ignore demographic factors completely by contending that these factors only marginally affect innate happiness level—a major index of subjective wellbeing as perceived by the current researcher.

Also examined were the relationships between five independent variables (i.e., self-efficacy, spirituality, social support, resilience, and leisure participation) and subjective wellbeing. Results showed there was a statistically significant relationship between the self-efficacy of respondents and their subjective wellbeing. The above finding was somewhat consistent with the results of research carried out by Bandura (1977, 1978, 1981, 1995, 1997). Bandura believed that establishing a connection between self-efficacy and caregiving could have realistic inferences for caregiver interventions. On the basis of the current study's finding, the first null hypothesis stating there would be no relationship between self-efficacy and subjective wellbeing of informal caregivers was rejected.

The results from the analysis of the independent variable of social support reflected a statistically significant relationship between respondents' social support and subjective wellbeing. Several scholars have noted that the resources from social support received by caregivers assist in reducing a host of negative outcomes (Williams et al., 2008). For example, Miller et al. (2001) suggested that the support received from informal networks alleviated the negative aspects of caregiving, such as emotional distress, health concerns, and economic strain. The results of the current study rejected the second null hypothesis stating there would be no relationship between social support and the subjective wellbeing of informal caregivers.

The findings of the current study align with the results of similar studies that depicted significant evidence of a substantial relationship between social support and caregivers' wellbeing (Atienza et al., 2001; Chang et al., 2001; Dilworth-Anderson et al., 2002; Franks & Stephens, 1996; Gerdner et al., 1996; Gupta & Pillai, 2000; Majerovitz, 2007; Pillemer & Suitor, 2002). Another study conducted by Franks and Stephens (1996) revealed that caregivers who had better emotional and social support generally reported decreased levels of depression and increased life satisfaction.

Similarly, Rapp et al. (1998) discovered that a caregiver's social resourcefulness and support he or she may receive from others were correlated with wellbeing. Gupta and Pillai (2000) came to a similar conclusion by suggesting that as a caregiver's social network expanded, his or her burden level decreased significantly. The current study further sustained this finding through the qualitative responses provided by the participants ($n = 28$) who perceived that a socially supportive environment encompassing family, friends, and the surrounding community was an essential ingredient in enhancing their ability to perform their caregiver responsibilities and maintaining their wellbeing.

There was no statistically significant relationship between the resilience of respondents and subjective wellbeing. Several researchers have defined resilience as an individual's ability to withstand obstacles and to persevere (Garity, 1997; Greene et al., 2002; Werner & Smith, 2001). This conclusion was expressed in other similar studies (Gaugler et al., 2000). There were some aspects of a study conducted by Ross et al. (2003) that revealed some relationship between a caregiver's resilience and subjective wellbeing. Ross et al. reported that caregivers who were deemed more resilient revealed several factors as most influential, including access to a good support system, appreciating the number of years as a caregiver, being physically active with hobbies, finding humor in a situation, staying spiritually connected, and maintaining their identity. There is little doubt that these perspectives, coupled with what the vast majority of the respondents ($n = 20$) in the current study believed as presented in the qualitative portion of the survey instrument, tend to contradict the results of the hypothesis testing, because most of the respondents, as suggested above, believed their resilience gave them a sense of optimism. Yet, on the basis of the correlation results of the current study, the third null hypothesis stating there would be no relationship between resilience and subjective wellbeing of informal caregivers failed to be rejected.

Conversely, results of the current study indicated there was a statistically significant relationship between the spirituality of the respondents and their subjective wellbeing. This result was also confirmed by the qualitative results ($n = 32$) in terms of respondents' perceptions of the relationship between their spiritual beliefs and their subjective wellbeing.

As confirmed by other empirical studies (Taylor, 2006; Tuck, 2004), and by the results of the correlation analyses conducted in this study, it appears there may exist a strong relationship between spirituality and subjective wellbeing. For example, Taylor (2006) and Tuck (2004) reported that a strong spiritual center is significant to individuals when confronted with highly stressful circumstances such as those involving an informal caregiver condition. Borrayo et al. (2007) reported that those who professed allegiance to God perceived their spiritual beliefs as having provided a source of strength in handling the challenges related to caregiving. Other scholars, such as Guberman et al. (1992) and Brotherson and Soderquist (2002), found that a positive relationship between caregivers and their religious beliefs enhanced their perception of their caring abilities. Hodge and Sun (2012) also identified a positive correlation between spirituality and caregiving. On the basis of the correlation results of the current study, the fourth null hypothesis stating there would be no relationship between spirituality and the subjective wellbeing of informal caregivers was rejected.

As noted previously, several studies have reinforced the notion that there may be a strong link between leisure participation and a caregiver's subjective wellbeing (Nieboer et al., 1998; Williamson et al., 1998). Wakui et al. (2012) intimated that a loss of leisure activities among caregivers may be closely linked to a host of deteriorating health issues such as increased depression and elevated levels of aggression. Staight and Harvey conducted research in 1990 that revealed an increase in depression scores among caregivers who attested to shortened session for relaxation. Studies conducted by other authors

(Gallagher-Thompson et al., 2000; Rivera et al., 1991) provided additional empirical evidence to indicate low levels of pleasant and social activities are associated with poorer caregiver wellbeing.

Last, results of the current study indicated there was a statistically significant relationship between the leisure participation of respondents and their subjective wellbeing. These findings were also confirmed by the qualitative responses given by the respondents ($n = 21$) as presented in Chapter 4. On the basis of this correlation finding the fifth null hypothesis stating there would be no relationship between leisure participation and the subjective wellbeing of informal caregivers was rejected

Concisely stated, the quantitative results yielded a rejection of the first null hypothesis stating there would be no relationship between self-efficacy and the subjective wellbeing of informal caregivers. Likewise, the second null hypothesis stating there would be no relationship between social support and the subjective wellbeing of informal caregivers was rejected. The third null hypothesis stating there would be no relationship between resilience and the subjective wellbeing of informal caregivers failed to be rejected. Additionally, the fourth null hypothesis stating there would be no relationship between spirituality and the subjective wellbeing of informal caregivers was rejected. It was also found that the fifth null hypothesis stating there would be no relationship between leisure participation and the subjective wellbeing of informal caregivers was rejected.

ASSESSMENT OF EMPIRICAL RESULTS AND IMPLICATIONS

One of the most significant findings of this study was that caregiving is often perceived by those who engage in it as an act of love. This suggests most informal caregivers may not necessarily be interested in pecuniary rewards for their efforts. Perhaps this is why the results showed that the gross income of informal caregivers was not necessarily a factor in enhancing their subjective wellbeing. Some of the relevant factors deemed most significant in enhancing subjective wellbeing were self-efficacy, social support, leisure participation, and spirituality. This proposition was supported by the results of prior studies (Borrayo et al., 2007; Gilliam & Steffen, 2006; Williamson et al., 1998).

The results of the current study revealed a strong link between self-efficacy and the subjective wellbeing of informal caregivers. A caregiver's ability to elevate his or her self-efficacy levels is critical to maintaining his or her own wellbeing (Farran et al., 2011; Kim & Given, 2008; Porter, Keefe, Garst, McBride, & Baucom, 2008). Accordingly, agencies that offer services to informal caregivers should consider objectives geared at improving their self-efficacy. Caregiver managers (commonly referred to as care managers), who are generally responsible for managing health care facilities, providing viable health care options for patients, and being advocates for the caregiver and care recipient, could also implement programs for informal caregivers that would advise them on the relevance of their own wellbeing. Such programs might focus specifically on teaching informal caregivers how to build confidence in their care-related skill sets. Caregivers could also be trained on the importance and development of self-care rituals and on how to create reasonable goals and outcomes, as well as learning to accept the inevitable occurrences of not exceeding all expectations yet embracing these experiences as constructive teaching moments.

Care managers might also consider offering another amenity such as the opportunity to expand a caregiver's social network or support system. This can occur by helping the caregiver to seek out both formal and informal support systems. Formal support systems comprise organizations such as daycare centers, respite services, and temporary or permanent residential facilities (Yang & Chen, 2008). Care managers can make objective recommendations for these facilities, assist with placement procedures, and aid in determining financial feasibility for the caregiver and care recipient.

Informal support comprises the caregiver's relationships with family members, friends, neighbors, and other individuals who interact with caregivers (Unger & Powell, 1980; Carlozzi et al, 2018). A care manager can arrange a cooperative meeting with those close to the informal caregiver to discuss how they can offer assistance. This would be beneficial to caregivers in helping them to alleviate some of the burdens often associated with their role and responsibilities as informal caregivers. This particular observation is consistent with some of the views expressed in the extant literature (Pillemer & Suitor, 2002; Rapp et al., 1998).

The current study also showed spirituality to be a major factor in understanding the psychological and sociological constitution of informal caregivers in terms of what elements contribute to their subjective wellbeing.

Thus, these caregivers believed their spirituality was important in aiding them to manage their responsibilities to the care recipient. Advocacy groups, medical institutions, social service agencies, religious leaders, public policymakers, and the general populace seeking to assist informal caregivers could also utilize this knowledge.

Given the fact that leisure participation was a strongly significant variable in terms of the factors that influence the subjective wellbeing of informal caregivers, it is proposed that it should become part of a frequent wellness regime. Oftentimes, the caregiver complains that lack of time impedes his or her pursuit of leisure time (Scharlach, 1994; Sisk, 2000). Care mangers can encourage caregiver participation in leisure activities by advising them of respite care options that might afford them more time to pursue personal interests.

The current study also showed continued involvement in leisure activities can positively influence caregivers' health. This claim is supported by various other studies on this topic. For example, the analytical objective of Pressman et al. (2009) was to determine whether engaging in various pleasurable activities was correlated with better psychological and physiological functioning. Their study involved a sample of 1,399 participants consisting of nearly 75% women between the ages of 19 and 89. The researchers utilized the self-report measure called the Pittsburgh Enjoyable Activities Test (PEAT). The results of the study showed that higher PEAT scores were associated with decreased blood pressure, reduced body mass index, reduced depression scores, and perceptions of improved physical functioning. The researchers concluded that caregivers who participated in a variety of leisure activities frequently experienced improved psychosocial and physical measurements relevant for good health. Pointedly, the researchers in the current study used a similar self-report measure and discovered that those participants who stated they regularly enjoyed leisure pursuits also expressed enhanced subjective wellbeing. These views were apparent in both the quantitative and qualitative analyses of the current study's survey responses.

It is evident that the act of caring for others will continue henceforth to be of primary consideration, just as it was for mankind several thousand years ago. The current study was designed to examine factors that might influence the subjective wellbeing of caregivers. Even though the current study was limited by its small sample size, the responses showed that self-efficacy, social support, spirituality, and leisure participation were viewed as critical components in enhancing a caregiver's subjective wellbeing. Although resilience was not shown to be significant based on the quantitative results, respondents claimed in their qualitative responses that it provided them a more optimistic attitude regarding their performance as caregivers. Also, several of the study respondents believed they were innately capable of handling their caregiving responsibilities. These views aligned with a fundamental aspect of Bandura's (1995) self-efficacy theory, which stresses that an individual's psychological presence affects how he or she perceives his or her abilities in different situations. This ultimately affects how the caregiver behaves during challenging circumstances. Conversely, social support was slated as significant via the extant literature and study respondents' replies. These respondents considered that a socially supportive environment was an essential ingredient in maintaining their subjective wellbeing. Additionally, although some respondents stated they had limited time for leisure, most recognized that participation in individual leisure interests was germane to maintaining their stamina as effective caregivers. The vast majority of respondents viewed their spirituality as the cornerstone in sustaining their wellbeing and supplying them with a tangible source of strength during their caregiving journey.

RECOMMENDATIONS FOR FUTURE RESEARCH

This chapter provided a discussion of the extent to which the subjective wellbeing of informal caregivers may be affected by an array of factors. However, as with any study of this nature, many questions were left unanswered, including questions such as discovering how the nature of the kinship relationship affected the attitudes of potential caregivers toward care recipients, or perhaps exploring whether or not the belief in a divine power affects a caregiver's confidence in his or her abilities. Additionally, unlike the current study that involved an exploration of the attitudes of 36 African American informal caregivers belonging to religious organizations, further research could be conducted to examine the attitudes of a larger sample size from more diverse ethnic and racial groups in terms of gauging factors that influence their subjective wellbeing as informal caregivers. Last, on the basis of these and other questions, new lines of empirical inquiry should be encouraged to examine the effects of implementing programs and public policies designed to assist informal caregivers.

REFERENCES

Atienza, A. A., Collins, R., & King, A. C. (2001). The mediating effects of situational control on social support and mood following a stressor: A prospective study of dementia caregivers in their natural environments. *The Journals of Gerontology. Series B, Psychological Sciences and Social Sciences*, *56*(3), S129–S139. doi:10.1093/geronb/56.3.S129 PMID:11316838

Bandura, A. (1977). Self-efficacy: Toward a unifying theory of behavioral change. *Psychological Review*, *84*(2), 191–215. doi:10.1037/0033-295X.84.2.191 PMID:847061

Bandura, A. (1978). Reflections on self-efficacy. In S. Rachman (Ed.), *Advances in behavior research and therapy* (pp. 237–269). Oxford, UK: Pergamon.

Bandura, A. (1981). Self-referent thought: A developmental analysis of self-efficacy. In J. H. Flavell & L. Ross (Eds.), *Social cognitive development: Frontiers and possible futures* (pp. 200–239). New York, NY: Cambridge University Press.

Bandura, A. (1995). Exercise of personal and collective efficacy in changing societies. *Self-Efficacy in Changing Societies*, *15*, 334.

Bandura, A. (1997). *Self-efficacy: The exercise of control*. New York, NY: W.H. Freeman and Company.

Borrayo, E. A., Goldwaser, G., Vacha-Haase, T., & Hepburn, K. W. (2007). An inquiry into Latino caregivers' experience caring for older adults with Alzheimer's disease and related dementias. *Journal of Applied Gerontology*, *26*(5), 486–505. doi:10.1177/0733464807305551

Brotherson, S. E., & Soderquist, J. (2002). Coping with a child's death: Spiritual issues and therapeutic implications. *Journal of Family Psychotherapy*, *13*(1-2), 53–86. doi:10.1300/J085v13n01_04

Carlozzi, N. E., Ianni, P. A., Tulsky, D. S., Brickell, T. A., Lange, R. T., French, L. M., ... Kratz, A. L. (2018). Understanding health-related quality of life in caregivers of civilians and service members/veterans with traumatic brain injury: Establishing the reliability and validity of PROMIS Fatigue and Sleep Disturbance item banks. *Archives of Physical Medicine and Rehabilitation*. PMID:29932884

Chang, B. L., Brecht, M. L., & Carter, P. A. (2001). Predictors of social support and caregiver outcomes. *Women & Health*, *33*(1-2), 39–61. doi:10.1300/J013v33n01_04 PMID:11523640

Cohen, C. A., Colantonio, A., & Vernich, L. (2002). Positive aspects of caregiving: Rounding out the caregiver experience. *International Journal of Geriatric Psychiatry*, *17*(2), 184–188. doi:10.1002/gps.561 PMID:11813283

Creswell, J. W. (2007). *Qualitative inquiry and research design: Choosing among five approaches* (2nd ed.). Thousand Oaks, CA: Sage.

Diener, E. (2000). Subjective wellbeing: The science of happiness and a proposal for a national index. *The American Psychologist*, *55*(1), 34–43. doi:10.1037/0003-066X.55.1.34 PMID:11392863

Diener, E., & Diener, C. (1996). Most people are happy. *Psychological Science*, *7*(3), 181–185. doi:10.1111/j.1467-9280.1996.tb00354.x PMID:11894851

Dilworth-Anderson, P., Williams, I. C., & Gibson, B. E. (2002). Issues of race, ethnicity, and culture in caregiving research: A 20-year review (1980–2000). *The Gerontologist*, *42*(2), 237–272. doi:10.1093/geront/42.2.237 PMID:11914467

Farran, C. J., Fogg, L. G., McCann, J. J., Etkin, C., Dong, X., & Barnes, L. L. (2011). Assessing family caregiver skill in managing behavioral symptoms of Alzheimer's disease. *Aging & Mental Health*, *15*(4), 510–521. doi:10.1080/13607863.2010.536140 PMID:21500018

Fluegel, J. C. (1925). A quantitative study of feeling and emotion in everyday life. *The British Journal of Psychology. General Section*, *15*(4), 318–355. doi:10.1111/j.2044-8295.1925.tb00187.x

Franks, M. M., & Stephens, M. A. P. (1996). Social support in the context of caregiving: Husbands' provision of support to wives involved in parent care. *The Journals of Gerontology. Series B, Psychological Sciences and Social Sciences*, *51*(1), 43–P52. doi:10.1093/geronb/51B.1.P43 PMID:8548517

Gallagher-Thompson, D., Aréan, P., Coon, D., Menendez, A., Takagi, K., Haley, W., & Szapocznik, J. (2000). Development and implementation of intervention strategies for culturally diverse caregiving populations. In R. Schulz (Ed.), *Handbook on dementia caregiving* (pp. 151–185). New York, NY: Springer.

Garity, J. (1997). Stress, learning style, resilience factors, and ways of coping in Alzheimer family caregivers. *American Journal of Alzheimer's Disease and Other Dementias*, *12*(4), 171–178. doi:10.1177/153331759701200405

Gaugler, J. E., Davey, A., Pearlin, L. I., & Zarit, S. H. (2000). Modeling caregiver adaptation over time: The longitudinal impact of behavior problems. *Psychology and Aging*, *15*(3), 437–450. doi:10.1037/0882-7974.15.3.437 PMID:11014707

Gaynor, S. E. (1988). *The effects of home care on elderly female caregivers* (Unpublished doctoral dissertation). Rush University, Chicago, IL.

Gerdner, L. A., Hall, G. R., & Buckwalter, K. C. (1996). Caregiver training for people with Alzheimer's based on a stress threshold model. *Image--the Journal of Nursing Scholarship*, *28*(3), 241–246. doi:10.1111/j.1547-5069.1996.tb00358.x PMID:8854546

Gilliam, C. M., & Steffen, A. M. (2006). The relationship between caregiving self-efficacy and depressive symptoms in dementia family caregivers. *Aging & Mental Health*, *10*(2), 79–86. doi:10.1080/13607860500310658 PMID:16517482

Greene, R. R., Conrad, A. P., Livingstone, N. C., Barton, W. H., Watkins, M. L., Blundo, R., & Riley, J. G. (2002). *An integrated approach to practice, policy, and research*. Washington, DC: NASW Press.

Guberman, N., Maheu, P., & Maillé, C. (1992). Women as family caregivers: Why do they care? *The Gerontologist*, *32*(5), 607–617. doi:10.1093/geront/32.5.607 PMID:1427272

Gupta, R., & Pillai, V. K. (2000). Caregiver burden in South Asian families: A systems theory perspective. *Journal of Ethnic & Cultural Diversity in Social Work*, *9*(1-2), 41–53. doi:10.1300/J051v09n01_03

Haley, W. E., LaMonde, L. A., Han, B., Burton, A. M., & Schonwetter, R. (2003). Predictors of depression and life satisfaction among spousal caregivers in hospice: Application of a stress process model. *Journal of Palliative Medicine*, *6*(2), 215–224. doi:10.1089/109662103764978461 PMID:12854938

Hodge, D. R., & Sun, F. (2012). Positive feelings of caregiving among Latino Alzheimer's family caregivers: Understanding the role of spirituality. *Aging & Mental Health, 16*(6), 689–698. doi:10.1080/13607863.2012.678481 PMID:22512416

Kim, Y., & Given, B. A. (2008). Quality of life of family caregivers of cancer survivors. *Cancer, 112*(S11), 2556–2568. doi:10.1002/cncr.23449 PMID:18428199

Majerovitz, D. S. (2007). Predictors of burden and depression among nursing home family caregivers. *Aging & Mental Health, 11*(3), 323–329. doi:10.1080/13607860600963380 PMID:17558583

Miller, B., Townsend, A., Carpenter, E., Montgomery, R. V., Stull, D., & Young, R. F. (2001). Social support and caregiver distress a replication analysis. *The Journals of Gerontology. Series B, Psychological Sciences and Social Sciences, 56*(4), S249–S256. doi:10.1093/geronb/56.4.S249 PMID:11445617

Nieboer, A. P., Schulz, R., Matthews, K. A., Scheier, M. F., Ormel, J., & Lindenberg, S. M. (1998). Spousal caregivers' activity restriction and depression: A model for changes over time. *Social Science & Medicine, 47*(9), 1361–1371. doi:10.1016/S0277-9536(98)00214-7 PMID:9783879

Pillemer, K., & Suitor, J. J. (2002). Peer support for Alzheimer's caregivers: Is it enough to make a difference? *Research on Aging, 24*(2), 171–192. doi:10.1177/0164027502242001

Porter, L. S., Keefe, F. J., Garst, J., McBride, C. M., & Baucom, D. (2008). Self-efficacy for managing pain, symptoms, and function in patients with lung cancer and their informal caregivers: Associations with symptoms and distress. *Pain, 137*(2), 306–315. doi:10.1016/j.pain.2007.09.010 PMID:17942229

Pressman, S. D., Matthews, K. A., Cohen, S., Martire, L. M., Scheier, M., Baum, A., & Schulz, R. (2009). Association of enjoyable leisure activities with psychological and physical wellbeing. *Psychosomatic Medicine, 71*(7), 725–732. doi:10.1097/PSY.0b013e3181ad7978 PMID:19592515

Rapp, S. R., Shumaker, S., Schmidt, S., Naughton, M., & Anderson, R. (1998). Social resourcefulness: Its relationship to social support and wellbeing among caregivers of dementia victims. *Aging & Mental Health*, *2*(1), 40–48. doi:10.1080/13607869856920

Rivera, P. A., Rose, J. M., Futterman, A., Lovett, S. B., & Gallagher-Thompson, D. (1991). Dimensions of perceived social support in clinically depressed and nondepressed female caregivers. *Psychology and Aging*, *6*(2), 232–237. doi:10.1037/0882-7974.6.2.232 PMID:1863392

Roberts, H., Halpin-Healy, C., McGinnis, R., & Noble, J. (2014). Museum-based creative arts programming is associated with less dementia patient apathy and better caregiver wellbeing. *Neurology*, *82*(10Supplement), 1–002.

Ross, L., Holliman, D., & Dixon, D. R. (2003). Resiliency in family caregivers: Implications for social work practice. *Journal of Gerontological Social Work*, *40*(3), 81–96. doi:10.1300/J083v40n03_07

Rudd, A. G., Wolfe, C. D., Tilling, K., & Beech, R. (1997). Randomized controlled trial to evaluate early discharge scheme for patients with stroke. *BMJ (Clinical Research Ed.)*, *315*(7115), 1039–1044. doi:10.1136/bmj.315.7115.1039 PMID:9366727

Scharlach, A. E. (1994). Caregiving and employment: Competing or complementary roles? *The Gerontologist*, *34*(3), 378–385. doi:10.1093/geront/34.3.378 PMID:8076880

Sisk, R. J. (2000). Caregiver burden and health promotion. *International Journal of Nursing Studies*, *37*(1), 37–43. doi:10.1016/S0020-7489(99)00053-X PMID:10687808

Staight, P. R., & Harvey, S. M. (1990). Caregiver burden: A comparison between elderly women as primary and secondary caregivers for their spouses. *Journal of Gerontological Social Work*, *15*(1-2), 89–104. doi:10.1300/J083v15n01_10

Taylor, E. J. (2006, July). Prevalence and associated factors of spiritual needs among patients with cancer and family caregivers. *Oncology Nursing Forum*, *33*(4), 729–735. doi:10.1188/06.ONF.729-735 PMID:16858453

Tuck, I. (2004). Development of a spirituality intervention to promote healing. *Journal of Theory Construction & Testing*, *8*(2).

Unger, D. G., & Powell, D. R. (1980). Supporting families under stress: The role of social networks. *Family Relations*, *29*(4), 566–574. doi:10.2307/584473

Wakui, T., Saito, T., Agree, E. M., & Kai, I. (2012). Effects of home, outside leisure, social, and peer activity on psychological health among Japanese family caregivers. *Aging & Mental Health*, *16*(4), 500–506. doi:10.1080/13607863.2011.644263 PMID:22360698

Werner, E. E., & Smith, R. S. (2001). *Journeys from childhood to midlife: Risk, resilience, and recovery*. Ithaca, NY: Cornell University Press.

Williams, S. W., Williams, C. S., Zimmerman, S., Munn, J., Dobbs, D., & Sloane, P. D. (2008). Emotional and physical health of informal caregivers of residents at the end of life: The role of social support. *The Journals of Gerontology. Series B, Psychological Sciences and Social Sciences*, *63*(3), S171–S183. doi:10.1093/geronb/63.3.S171 PMID:18559692

Williamson, G. M., Shaffer, D. R., & Schulz, R. (1998). Activity restriction and prior relationship history as contributors to mental health outcomes among middle-aged and older spousal caregivers. *Health Psychology*, *17*(2), 152–162. doi:10.1037/0278-6133.17.2.152 PMID:9548706

Yang, S. J., & Chen, I. Y. (2008). A social network-based system for supporting interactive collaboration in knowledge sharing over peer-to-peer network. *International Journal of Human-Computer Studies*, *66*(1), 36–50. doi:10.1016/j.ijhcs.2007.08.005

ADDITIONAL READING

Donelan, K., Hill, C. A., Hoffman, C., Scoles, K., Feldman, P. H., Levine, C., & Gould, D. (2002). Challenge to care: Informal caregivers in a changing health system. *Health Affairs*, *21*(4), 222–231. doi:10.1377/hlthaff.21.4.222 PMID:12117133

Kim, G., Allen, R. S., Wang, S. Y., Park, S., Perkins, E. A., & Parmelee, P. (2018). The Relation Between Multiple Informal Caregiving Roles and Subjective Physical and Mental Health Status Among Older Adults: Do Racial/Ethnic Differences Exist? *The Gerontologist*. doi:10.1093/geront/gnx196 PMID:29373738

Pinquart, M., & Sorenson, S. (2007). Correlates of physical health of informal caregivers: A meta-analysis. *Journal of Gerontology*, *62*(2), 126–137. doi:10.1093/geronb/62.2.P126 PMID:17379673

Sherifali, D., Ali, M. U., Ploeg, J., Markle-Reid, M., Valaitis, R., Bartholomew, A., ... McAiney, C. (2018). Impact of Internet-Based Interventions on Caregiver Mental Health: Systematic Review and Meta-Analysis. *Journal of Medical Internet Research*, *20*(7), e10668. doi:10.2196/10668 PMID:29970358

Chapter 5
Personal Reflection:
A Postscript

ABSTRACT

This chapter encompasses a reflective autobiographic account of the principal investigator, Dr. Ware, that plumbs the depths of what it means to be an informal caregiver for a family member or loved one. The chapter traces her steps as a caregiver for her late mother and the joys of personal fulfillment (positive sense of social wellbeing) and occasional travails associated with an individual stepping in this role. The author uses the independent variables in the study (subjective wellbeing, self-efficacy, spirituality, social support, resilience, and leisure participation) as lenses to discuss a reflective account of her idiosyncratic experiences in the context of her own family.

INTRODUCTION

Caregiving often calls us to lean into love we didn't know possible. (Speers & Walker, 2013)

The day this researcher had to make the tragic decision to remove my mother's leg was when I realized Mom (or life) would never be the same. You see, my sister was against the procedure stating *"Mom has too much pride for this Debbie. She wouldn't want this. If I am ever unable to make health care choices for myself, don't hang onto to me like this. Please just release me."* At the time neither she nor this researcher realized how prophetic her words would

DOI: 10.4018/978-1-5225-7452-1.ch005

come to be. Gangrene had invaded Mom's foot which had travelled into her bloodstream causing her leg to become infected. The doctors' explained that Mom's leg needed to be removed if we wanted her to live any longer. Mom wasn't capable of making her own wellbeing decisions and had bestowed this responsibility onto me (her eldest daughter). My sister didn't believe Mom would want any of her extremities removed from her body. She *declared "Mom would want to leave this earth precisely as she arrived. All four limbs intact"*. This researcher just couldn't phantom Mom leaving us simply because of an infected foot. So Sharon (my sister) left the ultimate decision to me stating *"It's your choice. I've said my piece. You are the oldest"*. Mom lived another 2 years afterwards battling dementia, cancer and other health challenges. So this researcher never regretted her decision. And mom never mentioned its absence. At the time mom drew her last breath, this researcher and her sister had been informal caregivers for 14 years.

The experience is what prompted this researcher to research factors contributing to the subjective wellbeing of informal caregiving. This topic eventually became the subject of her dissertation. This researcher was certain that the lived occurrences of this phenomena (informal caregiving) was of relevance to an audience broader than my immediate family. As one of the things which connects us as humankind, is our ability to relate and progress in character and conscience through the instances we share alike. This segment of the book is this researcher's brief reflection (along with related instances of several of the study participants) of these experiences via the selected variables. It is this researcher's hope that this personal reflection will empower readers in similar circumstances.

Subjective Well Being

I am determined to be cheerful and happy in whatever situation I may find myself. For I have learned that the greater part of our misery or unhappiness is determined not by our circumstances but by our disposition. – Martha Washington (1789)

The concept of subjective wellbeing (SWB) has been studied for centuries by academia, philosophers, scholars and religious leaders. The essence of the concept explains an individuals' own valuation of their happiness and satisfaction of life. The idea of SWB is *"subjective"* according to an individual's own affective reaction and cognitive judgment. Happiness is often used interchangeably with SWB. Yet, SWB considers satisfaction generally, and the sense of contentment to an individual's own standard.

The interest in SWB of caregivers has peaked as the world's aging population and recent advances in medicine have contributed to a surge in the need for informal caregivers. Yet, there is scant research that addresses the positive correlates of caregiving as told by the individuals experiencing this phenomenon. This particular study sought to expand awareness of the constructive factors that informal caregivers' claimed made a positive difference in their day to day life while embracing the role of custodian. SWB was the dependent variable in the study, the independent variables were leisure participation, resilience, self-efficacy, social support, and spirituality.

As this researcher reflect on her SWB she considered her mental wellbeing during this time period. The researcher had always been a happy and positive person. As the circumstances of life tendered challenges this researcher reflected on a proverbial phrase used by my grandmother (and mom) *"Baby when life tosses you lemons, get a pitcher, some sugar and make lemonade"*. So as the researcher began to brace for those lemons she maintained a positive demeanor. This mindset continued during the researcher's caregiver years. The researcher doesn't recall ever being in a state of serious depression throughout this experience. The researcher believes this is a direct result of the optimistic upbringing she experienced as a child.

The researcher was more saddened at the predicament of my mother's condition. Whenever we spoke about her desires she often commented that she wanted another chance to fulfill some of her lifelong goals. And although she knew that she was mentally and physically unable to return to her former lifestyle she spoke of returning to school, starting her own medical staffing agency, and us jointly purchasing property. The harsh reality that these desires never came to fruition for her still plague me today.

As the researcher continues to ponder her SWB during this experience she is able to empathize with the positive experiences mentioned by several of the participants from her research study whose comments regarding their wellbeing are listed as follows *"It gives me an ideal on how to live my life…" "Helping others as a caregiver gives a wonderful sense of accomplishment and satisfaction that you're helping others at a time when they need it most…" "Being a caregiver is such an honor. It gives me great joy…" "It makes me feel blessed to be able to take care of my dad. I believe this is what God intended me to do."* These sentiments mirror the researcher's feelings of contentment during this experience.

Self-Efficacy

It is our duty as human beings to proceed as though the limits of our capabilities do not exist. – Pierre Teilhard de Chardin (n.d.)

Self-efficacy, in its purest sense, is a person's own belief that he or she can accomplish a specific goal or task. This concept holds much significance to informal caregivers as they may encounter obstacles routinely associated with their position. A caregiver's self-efficacy quotient is significant to their confidence level in fulfilling their custodial roles. Arguably, those individuals with higher levels of self-efficacy may attest they feel more confident in their role as a caregiver. This claim supports the researcher's personal experience and those of the participants' in the study.

This researcher's idea of self-efficacy manifests itself in an *"I can do anything I set my mind to"* internal mantra. This belief allowed me to experience the caregiver role with optimism even during the most challenging times. As mom's dementia progressed she sometimes became combative. She might refuse to participate in activities of daily living, or chose to defecate (intentionally) in the tub during a bath, or become upset for no apparent reason. Yet, her resolve remained strong to continue caring for her mom even during the *'difficult days'*, understanding that often her mom's behavior was attributed to the disease and/or her medication.

The study participants discussed an equally tenacious attitude regarding their self-efficacy trait in their caregiver role. They exclaimed *"I am a leader and I'm quick on my feet so most problems in my environment don't faze me. I can take on any task"*. "*As a working full-time employee with taxing responsibilities the duties associated with caring for a dependent parent often seem daunting. Yet the experience has made me very capable in multitasking"*. *"My belief that I could handle this task comforts me in my role as a caregiver"*. *"I strongly believe my capabilities...help me perform the tasks required of me"*. *"I know I am capable and able to perform my task in the role. I believe when you are confident you perform well"*.

Spirituality

We are not human beings having a spiritual experience; we are spiritual beings having a human experience. – Pierre Teilhard de Chardin (n.d.)

There are many definitions of the concept spirituality. In its many dimensions, the general consensus could describe spirituality as any kind of meaningful activity that causes blissful experiences, internal self-analysis, and/or a search for the sacred. It expands the understanding of the intersection between all things alive or departed. This connection is the source and substance of every soul. It is best described as the alpha and omega of existence.

The researcher has never seen herself as a religious person. However, once she begins to explore religious organizations she identified more with the philosophy of spirituality in its general sense. This curiosity continuously nourished her soul with the insight it desired, concerning attaining a more enlightened understanding of our passions and purpose as human beings. As a caregiver the researcher's spirituality became more prominent as obstacles arose. It allowed her to care for my mom in a spirit of compassionate consciousness.

The researcher expected that spirituality would be the most prominently significant variable amongst her study participants. Although this assumption did not prove accurate, the participant remarks demonstrated how prolific their spirituality did impact their caregiver actions. *"Spirituality affects my beliefs and that impacts my role as a caregiver. It guides my daily decisions and lightens my heart". "My spirituality and faith in God and his word the Bible guide and direct me in my role as a caregiver". "As a caregiver, spirituality is so important. It is definitely what gets you through the day" My spirituality allows me to remain focused in his care, I believe that if I didn't rely on my spirituality, I honestly would've neglected his care more. Spirituality is a huge motivation for doing the right thing"*

Social Support

No one is useless in this world who lightens the burden of others. (Dickens, 1865)

There is limited (if any) dispute that receiving social support during distressing lived experiences is instrumental. This assertion is often ratified by a vast majority of informal caregivers as being consequential to sustaining their wellbeing. The support received from formal and/or casual networks can alleviate the adverse aspects of caregiving. Often it is simply the notion that either received or perceived support is available to the caregiver. The researcher's own caregiving experience substantiates this opinion.

The researcher is appreciative that her journey of caregiving was shared between herself and her sister. They provided mutual support for each other during this passage. It was also a comfort to know that others within our social network (family members and friends) were available to offer assistance whenever necessary. They never felt alone throughout the experience, as we had others (oftentimes going through similar situations) who through their boundless prayers, comforting words and/or deeds made this variable tangible. Several of the study participants expressed similar sentiments.

Their comments included; "*I believe that social support, my personality, and personal experience do impact my role as a caregiver. When my friends say encouraging words or I overhear the experiences from other family members and friends, I know that things will be okay. It is good to have people around you; then you are better with them.*" "*The more support you have, the better caregiver you can be.*" "*A dear friend has been a real help in directing me to handle major issues like getting social services and navigating the medical system. She has directed me to various resources to assist in caring for my elderly aunt. I know her support has been invaluable*". "*Other people give you another way of looking at a situation. This can impact your caregiving in a positive way.*" "*My sister and I are our own support system. My mom took excellent care of us and we're in this 100% taking care of her.*"

Resilience

Life doesn't get easier or more forgiving; we get stronger and more resilient. (Maraboli, 2009)

There are substantial recent research findings stating that the presence of resilience helps informal caregivers remain optimistic and/or decreases the mental strain often linked to their custodial experience. Several of these discoveries summarized that more resilient caregivers exhibit high levels of self-reliance, independence, and determination. They consistently sway toward the positive aspects of caregiving by negating the route of misery and mournfulness. The manifestation of the resilience trait during my personal caregiver experiences provided me a persistent pillar of fortitude necessary for the ever evolving role.

The researcher's resilience was elevated via the presence of other significant factors such as; appreciating the comical nature of experiences, embracing a supportive base, nourishing my mental and physical wellbeing, staying spirituality connected and maintaining my own identify. Her sister and her frequently rejuvenated our resilience shares via what we termed *'stress cleansing retreats'*. Their retreat could be as simple as an impromptu cup of afternoon tea, treating each other to a matinee, or partaking of a planned spa excursion. They were vividly aware that we had to maintain our own resilience and wellbeing so that we could provide mom with the same quality of care she gave us.

The study participants from this research chimed that; *"My resilience helps tremendously. Both my own ability to keep going when under tremendous stress and in my ability to encourage/support/motivate the person I am caring for...and other family and friends when needed". "As a caregiver sometimes I reflect on the past to build up my strength because it helps me to continue my role as a caretaker; knowing what this person has done for me during my childhood years". "I think my level of resilience affects my caregiving skills because I can separate my experiences, not take things personally, and then continue to treat her".*

Leisure Participation

If you are losing your leisure, Look out! You may be losing your soul. – Logan Pearsall Smith (n.d.)

The responsibilities of providing care can often be the precipice toward chaos to the informal caregivers' leisure lifestyle. Leisurely pursuits are often derailed and sometimes extinguished entirely because of the demands of caregiving. Yet, it is the participation by the caregiver of leisure activities that can offer substantial benefits by promoting positive feelings, and providing external (and internal) stimulation thru socialization. The types of leisureliness depend on individual preferences. Most significant is the continued participation of leisure to maintaining increased wellbeing levels in the caregiver.

Since the researcher shared caregiver responsibilities with her sister it was easier for each of us to pursue our leisure pursuits. This helped them to avoid the stagnant state oftentimes experienced by those responsible for the custodial duties of an individual in poor health. It also helped the m sustain positive wellbeing while servicing mom's needs. Oftentimes they included mom in these recreations as it allowed us to create enjoyable family occasions in familiar and new surroundings. This offered each of them the caring, comforting and coterie environment essential for their SWB, individually.

The study participants remarked *"Leisure activities like going to a concert, taking a short trip, or just hanging out does give me that extra push. Participation in these activities makes me return to caregiving fresh and ready to perform". "I try to take time and schedule time for leisure activities. I realize the leisure activities play a role in my wellbeing to give me joy and enjoyment, and to refresh me and reinvigorate me to continue as a whole person, a better caregiver". "It is very important that I take time for pleasurable leisure activities with loved ones. If I do not give myself that gift, I am a lot less able to be my best self. This shows up in my decision-making, interpersonal interactions, and quality of care I provide." "Leisure activities are important to keeping a balance in your life. I strive to create time for leisure activities as well as maintaining the support needed for my caregiver role".*

CONCLUSION

The researcher's fourteen year journey as a caregiver envelopes her with vivid memories of occurrences that encompass laughter, lively occasions, loss and unconditional love. Their mom graciously primed them for her transition. They each felt honored that God had given them such a stellar example of a mother who always exhibited unwavering adoration for them. Often sacrificing her own joy so that their childhood memories had as few painful moments as possible. So when that day arrived, her sister Sharon and her had had an opportunity to prepare themselves for the grieving stages and the laborious process of living life after the passing of their biggest cheerleader.

The variables this researcher associated with her caregiving experiences developed naturally. As she reflects on the constructs that helped her sustain a positive wellbeing demeanor throughout those years she can attribute it to several factors previously mentioned; foremost a sacred connection to her spirituality helped sustain her. This variable along with inbred resilience and self-efficacy traits, a stable social support network, and a commitment to leisurely pursuits offered instrumental avenues of escape from the travails often associated with the caregiving experience.

Yet, this researcher would proclaim as we continue living this thing called life on earth, sometimes we get side-swiped. The researcher hadn't even realized her sugar bowl was empty, when life dropped her directly under a ripened lemon tree in the midst of hurricane season. On a sunny weekday morning in early October, 2013 she received a call from her sister's employer. The woman said something about Sharon being transported via ambulance to the hospital. Once the researcher arrived there, the doctors told me Sharon had suffered a pontine hemorrhage. The family was advised that this was a dismal diagnosis with an even bleaker prognosis. Her best outcome would be a persistent vegetative state for the remainder of her days. She was 49 years of age. Sharon would never want to live life in limbo. So on October 19, 2013 the choice was made to free Sharon from her earthly body. There wasn't an opportunity for caregiving so we were left only with shredded shavings of heart and memories of days gone by.

It is this hope that her seasons of caretaking will prompt others to appreciate the value of their caregiving experience and *relish every living moment* of the time spent leaning into love you perhaps never even imagined possible.

Yes,

RELISH EVERY LIVING MOMENT!

RELISH EVERY LIVING MOMENT!

RELISH EVERY LIVING MOMENT!

REFERENCES

Dickens, C. (1865). *Doctor marigold.* Fredonia, NY: Fredonia Books.

Logan Pearsall Smith. (n.d.). *AZQuotes.com.* Retrieved May 27, 2018, from AZQuotes.com Web site: http://www.azquotes.com/quote/556212

Maraboli, S. (2009). *Life, the truth & being free.* Port Washington, NY: Better Today Publishing.

Pierre Teilhard de Chardin Quotes. (n.d.a). *BrainyQuote.com.* Retrieved May 27, 2018, from BrainyQuote.com Web site: https://www.brainyquote.com/quotes/pierre_teilhard_de_chardi_156693

Pierre Teilhard de Chardin Quotes. (n.d.b). *BrainyQuote.com*. Retrieved June 2, 2018, from BrainyQuote.com Web site: https://www.brainyquote.com/quotes/pierre_teilhard_de_chardi_156693

Speers, P., & Walker, T. (2013). *The inspired caregiver: finding joy while caring for those you love*. Seattle, WA: Createspace Independent Publishing Platform.

Washington, M. (n.d.). *Letter, Martha Washington to Mercy Otis Warren, December 26, 1789*. Martha Washington, Item #25. Retrieved from http://marthawashington.us/items/show/25

Appendix

APPENDIX A

Pre-Screening Questionnaire

Pre-Screening Questions

1. Are you 18 years of age or older?
   a. Yes____________
   b. No ________________

If prospective participant responded that they are 18 years of age of older continue to question 2. If not thank them for their time and the meeting will be terminated.

2. Would you agree to complete a survey about informal caregivers and factors influencing quality of life?
   a. Yes____________
   b. No ________________

If prospective participant responded affirmatively continue to question 3. If not thank them for their time and the meeting will be terminated.

3. Do you currently provide care to an individual requiring your help with their activities of daily living?
   a. Yes____________
   b. No ________________

If prospective participant responded affirmatively continue to question 4. If not thank them for their time and the meeting will be terminated.

4. How long have you provided care to this individual?
   a. ______________ months
   b. ________________ years

If greater than 3 months then continue to question 4. If less than 3 months thank them for their time and the meeting will be terminated.

5. On a scale from 1 (not difficult at all) to 5 (extremely difficult) please indicate how difficult it would be for you to complete a survey regarding your caregiving experience.
   1. Not difficult at all
   2. Somewhat difficult
   3. Natural
   4. Very difficult
   5. Extremely difficult

If the individual selects a number from 1 to 3 on the grid (above) they will be eligible for the study.

If the prospective participant selects numbers 4 or 5 on the grid (above) they will be thanked for their time and the meeting will be terminated.

APPENDIX B

Survey Instrument

Questionnaire for informal caregivers instructions: Please read each question carefully and check the response which most accurately reflects your views.

1. Male_____ Female_____
2. Age:
   a. 18-35
   b. 36-45
   c. 46-55
   d. 56-65
   e. 66-75
   f. 75+
3. Race:
   a. African American/Black
   b. Alaska Native
   c. American Indian
   d. Asian
   e. Hispanic
   f. Native Hawaiian
   g. Pacific Islander
   h. White
   i. Other
4. Gross Household Income (2014)
   a. <$15,000
   b. $15,000 - $30,000
   c. $31,000 - $60,000
   d. $61,000 – $90,000
   e. $91,0000 - $120,000
   f. $121,000 - $150,000
   g. $151,000 +
5. (Average weekly hours providing care)
   a. < 1 hour
   b. 1 – 2 hours
   c. 3 – 6 hours
   d. 7 – 12 hours

e. > 12 hours

6. Caring Relationship (Who are you caring for – Circle all that apply)
   a. Parent
   b. Spouse
   c. Child
   d. Adult Offspring
   e. Grandchild
   f. Friend
   g. Neighbor
   h. Other
   i. Multiple individuals
7. How long have you been a care giver for the care recipient?
   a. ____________________ months
   b. ______________________ years
8. Type of Disability
   a. Chronic condition
   b. Mental illness
   c. Physical disability
   d. Aged & Frail
   e. Multiple disabilities
   f. Other

The following questions ask how satisfied you feel, on a scale from 10 to 0. Ten (10) means you feel completely satisfied and Zero (0) means you feel no satisfaction at all.

9. "Thinking about your own life and personal circumstances, overall how satisfied are you **with your life as a whole?**
   10 (Completely satisfied)
   9
   8
   7
   6
   5
   4
   3
   2
   1
   0 (No satisfaction at all)

10. "Overall, how satisfied are you **with your standard of living?"**
    10 (Completely satisfied)
    9
    8
    7
    6
    5
    4
    3
    2
    1
    0 (No satisfaction at all)
11. "Overall, how satisfied are you **with your health?"**
    10 (Completely satisfied)
    9
    8
    7
    6
    5
    4
    3
    2
    1
    0 (No satisfaction at all)
12. "Overall, how satisfied are you **with what you are achieving in life?"**
    10 (Completely satisfied)
    9
    8
    7
    6
    5
    4
    3
    2
    1
    0 (No satisfaction at all)

13.“Overall, how satisfied are you **with your personal relationships?”**
10 (Completely satisfied)
9
8
7
6
5
4
3
2
1
0 (No satisfaction at all)

14. “Overall, how satisfied are you **with how safe you feel?”**
10 (Completely satisfied)
9
8
7
6
5
4
3
2
1
0 (No satisfaction at all)

15. “Overall, how satisfied are you **with feeling part of your community?”**
10 (Completely satisfied)
9
8
7
6
5
4
3
2
1
0 (No satisfaction at all)

16. "Overall, how satisfied are you **with your future security?"**
    10 (Completely satisfied)
    9
    8
    7
    6
    5
    4
    3
    2
    1
    0 (No satisfaction at all)

Briefly explain how your role as a caregiver affects your ability to maintain a quality of life you desire?

____
____
____
____
____

Please indicate the extent to which you agree with each of the following statements by selecting the numbered box adjacent to the text which represents your view.

17. I can always mange to solve difficult problems if I try hard enough.
    1 = Strongly agree
    2 = Agree
    3 = Neutral
    4 = Disagree
    5 = Strongly disagree
18. If someone opposes me, I can find the means and ways to get what I want.
    1 = Strongly agree
    2 = Agree
    3 = Neutral
    4 = Disagree
    5 = Strongly disagree

19. It is easy for me to stick to my aims and accomplish my goals.
    1 = Strongly agree
    2 = Agree
    3 = Neutral
    4 = Disagree
    5 = Strongly disagree
20. I am confident that I could deal efficiently with unexpected events.
    1 = Strongly agree
    2 = Agree
    3 = Neutral
    4 = Disagree
    5 = Strongly disagree
21. Thanks to my resourcefulness, I know how to handle unforeseen situations.
    1 = Strongly agree
    2 = Agree
    3 = Neutral
    4 = Disagree
    5 = Strongly disagree
22. I can solve most problems if I invest the necessary effort.
    1 = Strongly agree
    2 = Agree
    3 = Neutral
    4 = Disagree
    5 = Strongly disagree
23. I can remain calm when facing difficulties because I can rely on my coping abilities.
    1 = Strongly agree
    2 = Agree
    3 = Neutral
    4 = Disagree
    5 = Strongly disagree
24. When I am confronted with a problem, I can usually find several solutions.
    1 = Strongly agree
    2 = Agree
    3 = Neutral
    4 = Disagree
    5 = Strongly disagree

25. If I am in trouble, I can usually think of a solution.
    1 = Strongly agree
    2 = Agree
    3 = Neutral
    4 = Disagree
    5 = Strongly disagree
26. I can usually handle whatever comes my way.
    1 = Strongly agree
    2 = Agree
    3 = Neutral
    4 = Disagree
    5 = Strongly disagree

Briefly explain how your belief in your capabilities as a caregiver impacts your responsibilities in that role? (Please print)

____

____

____

____

____

27. There is a special person who is around when I am in need.
    1 = Strongly agree
    2 = Agree
    3 = Neutral
    4 = Disagree
    5 = Strongly disagree
28. There is a special person with whom I can share my joys and sorrows.
    1 = Strongly agree
    2 = Agree
    3 = Neutral
    4 = Disagree
    5 = Strongly disagree
29. My family really tries to help me.
    1 = Strongly agree
    2 = Agree
    3 = Neutral
    4 = Disagree
    5 = Strongly disagree

30. I get the emotional help and support I need from my family.
    1 = Strongly agree
    2 = Agree
    3 = Neutral
    4 = Disagree
    5 = Strongly disagree
31. I have a special person who is a real source of comfort to me.
    1 = Strongly agree
    2 = Agree
    3 = Neutral
    4 = Disagree
    5 = Strongly disagree
32. My friends really try to help me.
    1 = Strongly agree
    2 = Agree
    3 = Neutral
    4 = Disagree
    5 = Strongly disagree
33. I can count on my friends when things go wrong.
    1 = Strongly agree
    2 = Agree
    3 = Neutral
    4 = Disagree
    5 = Strongly disagree
34. I can talk about my problems with my family.
    1 = Strongly agree
    2 = Agree
    3 = Neutral
    4 = Disagree
    5 = Strongly disagree
35. I have friends with whom I can share my joys and sorrows.
    1 = Strongly agree
    2 = Agree
    3 = Neutral
    4 = Disagree
    5 = Strongly disagree

36. There is a special person in my life who cares about my feelings.
    1 = Strongly agree
    2 = Agree
    3 = Neutral
    4 = Disagree
    5 = Strongly disagree
37. My family is willing to help me make decisions.
    1 = Strongly agree
    2 = Agree
    3 = Neutral
    4 = Disagree
    5 = Strongly disagree
38. I can talk about my problems with my friends.
    1 = Strongly agree
    2 = Agree
    3 = Neutral
    4 = Disagree
    5 = Strongly disagree

Briefly explain how support from other people impacts your role as a caregiver? (Please print)

____

____

____

____

____

____

39. I tend to bounce back quickly after hard times.
    1 = Strongly agree
    2 = Agree
    3 = Neutral
    4 = Disagree
    5 = Strongly disagree
40. I have a hard time making it through stressful events.
    1 = Strongly agree
    2 = Agree
    3 = Neutral
    4 = Disagree
    5 = Strongly disagree

41. It does not take me long to recover from a stressful event.
    1 = Strongly agree
    2 = Agree
    3 = Neutral
    4 = Disagree
    5 = Strongly disagree
42. It is hard for me to snap back when something bad happens.
    1 = Strongly agree
    2 = Agree
    3 = Neutral
    4 = Disagree
    5 = Strongly disagree
43. I usually come through difficult times with little trouble.
    1 = Strongly agree
    2 = Agree
    3 = Neutral
    4 = Disagree
    5 = Strongly disagree
44. I tend to take a long time to get over set-backs in my life.
    1 = Strongly agree
    2 = Agree
    3 = Neutral
    4 = Disagree
    5 = Strongly disagree

Briefly explain how your level of resilience affects your role as a caregiver?

____

____

____

____

____

____

Please indicate the extent to which you agree with each of the following statements by selecting the number closest to the statement which represents how you feel.

45. In terms of the questions I have about life:
    10 (My spirituality answers all my questions)
    9
    8
    7
    6
    5
    4
    3
    2
    1
    0 My spirituality answers no questions
46. Growing spirituality is:
    10 (More important than anything else in my life)
    9
    8
    7
    6
    5
    4
    3
    2
    1
    0 (Of no importance in my life to me)
47. When I am faced with an important decision my spirituality:
    10 (It is the overriding consideration)
    9
    8
    7
    6
    5
    4
    3
    2
    1
    0 (Plays absolutely no role)

48. Spirituality is:
    10 (The master motive of my life, directing every other aspect of my life)
    9
    8
    7
    6
    5
    4
    3
    2
    1
    0 (Not part of my life)
49. When I think of things that help me to grow and mature as a person, my spirituality:
    10 (Is absolutely the most important factor in my personal growth)
    9
    8
    7
    6
    5
    4
    3
    2
    1
    0 (Has no effect on my personal growth)
50. My spiritual beliefs affect:
    10 (Absolutely every aspect of my life)
    9
    8
    7
    6
    5
    4
    3
    2
    1
    0 (No aspect of my life)

Briefly explain how your spirituality affects your role as a caregiver. (Please print)

____

____

____

____

____

____

____

Please indicate the extent to which you agree with each of the following statements by selecting the number below the response which represents how you feel.

Over the past month, how satisfied are you with amount of time you have been able to spend:

51. In quiet time by yourself?
    2 (A lot)
    1 (A little)
    0 (Not at all)
52. Attending church or going to other meetings of groups or organization?
    2 (A lot)
    1 (A little)
    0 (Not at all)
53. Taking part in hobbies or other interests?
    2 (A lot)
    1 (A little)
    0 (Not at all)
54. Going out for meals or other social activities?
    2 (A lot)
    1 (A little)
    0 (Not at all)
55. Doing fun things with other people?
    2 (A lot)
    1 (A little)
    0 (Not at all)
56. Visiting with family and friends?
    2 (A lot)
    1 (A little)
    0 (Not at all)

Briefly explain how important your participation in leisure activities (if any) affects your ability as a caregiver. (Please print)

____

____

____

____

____

____

Related Readings

To continue IGI Global's long-standing tradition of advancing innovation through emerging research, please find below a compiled list of recommended IGI Global book chapters and journal articles in the areas of caregiving, mental illness, and home nursing. These related readings will provide additional information and guidance to further enrich your knowledge and assist you with your own research.

Ahmmed, F. (2018). Gender Dimensions of Aging Among Indigenous People: A Case Study on Khasi Indigenous Group in Bangladesh. In R. Pande & T. van der Weide (Eds.), *Handbook of Research on Multicultural Perspectives on Gender and Aging* (pp. 142–158). Hershey, PA: IGI Global. doi:10.4018/978-1-5225-4772-3.ch011

Akbar, S., & Khurana, H. (2017). Chronic Mental Illness in Old Age Homes: An International Perspective. In B. Prasad (Ed.), *Chronic Mental Illness and the Changing Scope of Intervention Strategies, Diagnosis, and Treatment* (pp. 21–39). Hershey, PA: IGI Global. doi:10.4018/978-1-5225-0519-8.ch002

Amor, J., & James, C. (2015). Unobtrusive Wearable Technology for Health Monitoring. In P. Bamidis, I. Tarnanas, L. Hadjileontiadis, & M. Tsolaki (Eds.), *Handbook of Research on Innovations in the Diagnosis and Treatment of Dementia* (pp. 382–395). Hershey, PA: IGI Global. doi:10.4018/978-1-4666-8234-4.ch020

Antoniou, P. E., Konstantinidis, E., Billis, A. S., Bamparopoulos, G., Tsatali, M. S., & Sioundas, A. (2015). Instrumenting the eHome and Preparing Elderly Pilots: The USEFIL Approach. In P. Bamidis, I. Tarnanas, L. Hadjileontiadis, & M. Tsolaki (Eds.), *Handbook of Research on Innovations in the Diagnosis and Treatment of Dementia* (pp. 335–361). Hershey, PA: IGI Global. doi:10.4018/978-1-4666-8234-4.ch018

Astaras, A. (2015). Graceful Ageing: Exergaming as a Means to Delay Mental and Physical Decline among the Elderly. In P. Bamidis, I. Tarnanas, L. Hadjileontiadis, & M. Tsolaki (Eds.), *Handbook of Research on Innovations in the Diagnosis and Treatment of Dementia* (pp. 37–46). Hershey, PA: IGI Global. doi:10.4018/978-1-4666-8234-4.ch003

Astaras, A., Lewy, H., James, C., Katasonov, A., Ruschin, D., & Bamidis, P. D. (2015). Unobtrusive Smart Environments for Independent Living and the role of Mixed Methods in Elderly Healthcare Delivery: The USEFIL Approach. In P. Bamidis, I. Tarnanas, L. Hadjileontiadis, & M. Tsolaki (Eds.), *Handbook of Research on Innovations in the Diagnosis and Treatment of Dementia* (pp. 290–305). Hershey, PA: IGI Global. doi:10.4018/978-1-4666-8234-4.ch015

B. N. R., Prasad, B. V., & Tavaragi, M. S. (2017). Legal Aspects of Chronic Mental Illness. In B. Prasad (Ed.), Chronic Mental Illness and the Changing Scope of Intervention Strategies, Diagnosis, and Treatment (pp. 225-235). Hershey, PA: IGI Global. doi:10.4018/978-1-5225-0519-8.ch012

Bamidis, P. D., Konstantinidis, E., Billis, A. S., & Sioundas, A. (2015). Reviewing Home Based Assistive Technologies. In P. Bamidis, I. Tarnanas, L. Hadjileontiadis, & M. Tsolaki (Eds.), *Handbook of Research on Innovations in the Diagnosis and Treatment of Dementia* (pp. 317–334). Hershey, PA: IGI Global. doi:10.4018/978-1-4666-8234-4.ch017

Bandila, R. K. (2018). Concerns of Elderly Women's Wellbeing: Some Policy Issues. In R. Pande & T. van der Weide (Eds.), *Handbook of Research on Multicultural Perspectives on Gender and Aging* (pp. 231–240). Hershey, PA: IGI Global. doi:10.4018/978-1-5225-4772-3.ch017

Beard, R. L., & O'Connor, M. K. (2015). Listening to Alzheimer's: The Role of Social Location in Illness Narratives. In C. Dick-Muehlke, R. Li, & M. Orleans (Eds.), *Psychosocial Studies of the Individual's Changing Perspectives in Alzheimer's Disease* (pp. 1–32). Hershey, PA: IGI Global. doi:10.4018/978-1-4666-8478-2.ch001

Bedi, D. (2017). Efficacy of Art Therapy in Treating Patients with Paranoid Schizophrenia. In B. Prasad (Ed.), *Chronic Mental Illness and the Changing Scope of Intervention Strategies, Diagnosis, and Treatment* (pp. 308–320). Hershey, PA: IGI Global. doi:10.4018/978-1-5225-0519-8.ch017

Behrani, P., & Deka, D. B. (2016). Concerns for Individuals with Intellectual Disability in India. In R. Gopalan (Ed.), *Handbook of Research on Diagnosing, Treating, and Managing Intellectual Disabilities* (pp. 204–219). Hershey, PA: IGI Global. doi:10.4018/978-1-5225-0089-6.ch011

Bender, S., & Hill, K. (2018). Special Issue: Sexually Transmitted Infections – Diagnoses, Stigma, and Mental Health. In B. Canfield & H. Cunningham (Eds.), *Deconstructing Stigma in Mental Health* (pp. 184–208). Hershey, PA: IGI Global. doi:10.4018/978-1-5225-3808-0.ch008

Bezbaruah, V., & Mehrotra, N. (2018). Gendered Understanding of Disability and Aging: A North Indian Context. In R. Pande & T. van der Weide (Eds.), *Handbook of Research on Multicultural Perspectives on Gender and Aging* (pp. 241–253). Hershey, PA: IGI Global. doi:10.4018/978-1-5225-4772-3.ch018

Bhargava, S., & Umrigar, D. M. (2016). Intellectual Disability in the Family Context: Parents with Intellectual Disability. In R. Gopalan (Ed.), *Handbook of Research on Diagnosing, Treating, and Managing Intellectual Disabilities* (pp. 370–385). Hershey, PA: IGI Global. doi:10.4018/978-1-5225-0089-6.ch019

Billingsley, K. Y., & Corey, D. R. (2018). Deconstructing Racial Stigma in the Therapeutic Relationship. In B. Canfield & H. Cunningham (Eds.), *Deconstructing Stigma in Mental Health* (pp. 1–19). Hershey, PA: IGI Global. doi:10.4018/978-1-5225-3808-0.ch001

Billis, A. S., Frantzidis, C. A., & Bamidis, P. D. (2015). Decision Support in the Elderly Healthcare: Combing Short- and Long-Term Analysis Aspects. In P. Bamidis, I. Tarnanas, L. Hadjileontiadis, & M. Tsolaki (Eds.), *Handbook of Research on Innovations in the Diagnosis and Treatment of Dementia* (pp. 175–195). Hershey, PA: IGI Global. doi:10.4018/978-1-4666-8234-4.ch010

Bosco, N., Giaccherini, S., Petrini, F., Castagnoli, S., & Meringolo, P. (2018). Fighting Stigma in the Community: Bridging Ties Through Social Innovation Interventions. In B. Canfield & H. Cunningham (Eds.), *Deconstructing Stigma in Mental Health* (pp. 133–168). Hershey, PA: IGI Global. doi:10.4018/978-1-5225-3808-0.ch006

Card, S., & Wang, H. (2015). Taking Care to Play: Meaningful Communication in Dementia Care in Chinese Culture. In C. Dick-Muehlke, R. Li, & M. Orleans (Eds.), *Psychosocial Studies of the Individual's Changing Perspectives in Alzheimer's Disease* (pp. 76–103). Hershey, PA: IGI Global. doi:10.4018/978-1-4666-8478-2.ch004

Chaldogeridis, A., Kyropoulou, K., Malegiannaki, A., Nikolaidou, E., & Tsiatsos, T. (2015). Implementing Cognitive Exercises in Electronic Form for Supporting Patients with Alzheimer's Disease: The Greek Case. In P. Bamidis, I. Tarnanas, L. Hadjileontiadis, & M. Tsolaki (Eds.), *Handbook of Research on Innovations in the Diagnosis and Treatment of Dementia* (pp. 130–146). Hershey, PA: IGI Global. doi:10.4018/978-1-4666-8234-4.ch007

Chan, E., Seto, S. W., Au Yeung, T. M., & Chan, G. H. (2018). Chinese Herbal Medicine in the Management of Atherosclerosis-Related Chronic Conditions in an Aging Population. In B. Fong, A. Ng, & P. Yuen (Eds.), *Sustainable Health and Long-Term Care Solutions for an Aging Population* (pp. 320–342). Hershey, PA: IGI Global. doi:10.4018/978-1-5225-2633-9.ch017

Cheung, S. T., & Dawkes, S. (2018). Eating Habits of Young Persons for Healthy Aging: An Exploratory Study Involving University Students in Hong Kong. In B. Fong, A. Ng, & P. Yuen (Eds.), *Sustainable Health and Long-Term Care Solutions for an Aging Population* (pp. 343–356). Hershey, PA: IGI Global. doi:10.4018/978-1-5225-2633-9.ch018

Chowhan, S., & Patowary, P. (2016). Issues and Recent Trends in the Assessment and Management of ID in Childhood. In R. Gopalan (Ed.), *Handbook of Research on Diagnosing, Treating, and Managing Intellectual Disabilities* (pp. 186–203). Hershey, PA: IGI Global. doi:10.4018/978-1-5225-0089-6.ch010

Davidson, T., Moreland, A., Bunnell, B. E., Winkelmann, J., Hamblen, J. L., & Ruggiero, K. J. (2018). Reducing Stigma in Mental Health Through Digital Storytelling. In B. Canfield & H. Cunningham (Eds.), *Deconstructing Stigma in Mental Health* (pp. 169–183). Hershey, PA: IGI Global. doi:10.4018/978-1-5225-3808-0.ch007

Dawkes, S., & Cheung, S. T. (2018). United Kingdom Health Promotion Initiatives for Healthy Aging. In B. Fong, A. Ng, & P. Yuen (Eds.), *Sustainable Health and Long-Term Care Solutions for an Aging Population* (pp. 91–102). Hershey, PA: IGI Global. doi:10.4018/978-1-5225-2633-9.ch005

Dehuri, B. K., & Mukund, B. (2016). Recent Trends and Issues in Vocational Rehabilitation of People with ID. In R. Gopalan (Ed.), *Handbook of Research on Diagnosing, Treating, and Managing Intellectual Disabilities* (pp. 283–309). Hershey, PA: IGI Global. doi:10.4018/978-1-5225-0089-6.ch015

Demetriadis, S., Giannouli, V., & Sapounidis, T. (2015). Robot Programming and Tangible Interfaces for Cognitive Training. In P. Bamidis, I. Tarnanas, L. Hadjileontiadis, & M. Tsolaki (Eds.), *Handbook of Research on Innovations in the Diagnosis and Treatment of Dementia* (pp. 196–223). Hershey, PA: IGI Global. doi:10.4018/978-1-4666-8234-4.ch011

Eapen, V., & Walter, A. (2016). Mind the Gap: Developmental Vulnerability and Mental Health. In R. Gopalan (Ed.), *Handbook of Research on Diagnosing, Treating, and Managing Intellectual Disabilities* (pp. 11–32). Hershey, PA: IGI Global. doi:10.4018/978-1-5225-0089-6.ch002

Fazio, S., & Mitchell, D. B. (2015). Self-Preservation in Individuals with Alzheimer's Disease: Empirical Evidence and the Role of the Social Environment. In C. Dick-Muehlke, R. Li, & M. Orleans (Eds.), *Psychosocial Studies of the Individual's Changing Perspectives in Alzheimer's Disease* (pp. 183–207). Hershey, PA: IGI Global. doi:10.4018/978-1-4666-8478-2.ch008

Firdaus, J., & Jadeja, M. (2016). Quality of Life of People with Intellectual Disability. In R. Gopalan (Ed.), *Handbook of Research on Diagnosing, Treating, and Managing Intellectual Disabilities* (pp. 139–155). Hershey, PA: IGI Global. doi:10.4018/978-1-5225-0089-6.ch008

Fong, B. Y., & Law, V. T. (2018). Aging in Place. In B. Fong, A. Ng, & P. Yuen (Eds.), *Sustainable Health and Long-Term Care Solutions for an Aging Population* (pp. 259–276). Hershey, PA: IGI Global. doi:10.4018/978-1-5225-2633-9.ch014

Freitas, M. H., Fukuda, C. C., Alves, V. P., & Gomes, L. D. (2018). Religiosity and Attitude in the Face of Death in Brazilian Elderly. In R. Pande & T. van der Weide (Eds.), *Handbook of Research on Multicultural Perspectives on Gender and Aging* (pp. 126–141). Hershey, PA: IGI Global. doi:10.4018/978-1-5225-4772-3.ch010

G., L. (2017). Psychosocial Intervention Studies for Street Children with Substance Abuse. In B. Prasad (Ed.), *Chronic Mental Illness and the Changing Scope of Intervention Strategies, Diagnosis, and Treatment* (pp. 237-257). Hershey, PA: IGI Global. doi:10.4018/978-1-5225-0519-8.ch013

Galvin, J. E., & Kelleher, M. E. (2015). Dementia and Other Neurocognitive Disorders: An Overview. In C. Dick-Muehlke, R. Li, & M. Orleans (Eds.), *Psychosocial Studies of the Individual's Changing Perspectives in Alzheimer's Disease* (pp. 104–130). Hershey, PA: IGI Global. doi:10.4018/978-1-4666-8478-2.ch005

Garg, B., Khanna, P., & Khanna, A. (2017). Chronic Mental Illness and the Changing Scope of Intervention Strategies, Diagnosis, and Treatment in Child and Adolescent Population. In B. Prasad (Ed.), *Chronic Mental Illness and the Changing Scope of Intervention Strategies, Diagnosis, and Treatment* (pp. 258–269). Hershey, PA: IGI Global. doi:10.4018/978-1-5225-0519-8.ch014

Georgakopoulos, P., Chatzidimitriou, M., & Tsolaki, M. (2015). A Review of Interventions with Assistive Technologies for Patients with Cognitive Impairment. In P. Bamidis, I. Tarnanas, L. Hadjileontiadis, & M. Tsolaki (Eds.), *Handbook of Research on Innovations in the Diagnosis and Treatment of Dementia* (pp. 118–129). Hershey, PA: IGI Global. doi:10.4018/978-1-4666-8234-4.ch006

Ghosh, N., Sinha, V. K., & Poddar, S. (2016). Vocational Rehabilitation: Recent Trends and Issues in Vocational Rehabilitation of People with ID. In R. Gopalan (Ed.), *Handbook of Research on Diagnosing, Treating, and Managing Intellectual Disabilities* (pp. 310–330). Hershey, PA: IGI Global. doi:10.4018/978-1-5225-0089-6.ch016

Ghosh, S. (2018). Quality of Life and Aging of Women. In R. Pande & T. van der Weide (Eds.), *Handbook of Research on Multicultural Perspectives on Gender and Aging* (pp. 1–10). Hershey, PA: IGI Global. doi:10.4018/978-1-5225-4772-3.ch001

Giannouli, V. (2016). Crime and Legal Issues among Intellectually Disabled Individuals. In R. Gopalan (Ed.), *Handbook of Research on Diagnosing, Treating, and Managing Intellectual Disabilities* (pp. 346–369). Hershey, PA: IGI Global. doi:10.4018/978-1-5225-0089-6.ch018

Gök, F. A., & Çifci, E. G. (2018). Stamped Life: Stigmatization Stories of Women Who Care for Patients With Schizophrenia. In B. Canfield & H. Cunningham (Eds.), *Deconstructing Stigma in Mental Health* (pp. 209–224). Hershey, PA: IGI Global. doi:10.4018/978-1-5225-3808-0.ch009

Gopalan, R. T. (2016). Intellectual Disability: From History to Recent Trends. In R. Gopalan (Ed.), *Handbook of Research on Diagnosing, Treating, and Managing Intellectual Disabilities* (pp. 1–10). Hershey, PA: IGI Global. doi:10.4018/978-1-5225-0089-6.ch001

Gopalan, R. T., & Agustus, P. (2016). Sexuality, Parenting Skills, and Related Issues in Persons with Intellectual Disability. In R. Gopalan (Ed.), *Handbook of Research on Diagnosing, Treating, and Managing Intellectual Disabilities* (pp. 386–395). Hershey, PA: IGI Global. doi:10.4018/978-1-5225-0089-6.ch020

Gupta, N., & Raju, S. S. (2018). Policies, Programs, and Schemes for the Elderly in India: A Critical Review. In R. Pande & T. van der Weide (Eds.), *Handbook of Research on Multicultural Perspectives on Gender and Aging* (pp. 11–25). Hershey, PA: IGI Global. doi:10.4018/978-1-5225-4772-3.ch002

Gupta, S. K. (2016). Use of Assistive Technology to Empower Persons with Intellectual Disabilities. In R. Gopalan (Ed.), *Handbook of Research on Diagnosing, Treating, and Managing Intellectual Disabilities* (pp. 331–345). Hershey, PA: IGI Global. doi:10.4018/978-1-5225-0089-6.ch017

Hadjileontiadis, L. J., Mandiliotis, D., Toumpas, K., & Kyprioti, A. (2015). Towards an HCI-Based Symbiotic Environment for Alzheimer's Support. In P. Bamidis, I. Tarnanas, L. Hadjileontiadis, & M. Tsolaki (Eds.), *Handbook of Research on Innovations in the Diagnosis and Treatment of Dementia* (pp. 240–268). Hershey, PA: IGI Global. doi:10.4018/978-1-4666-8234-4.ch013

Halder, S., & Mahato, A. (2017). Cognitive Remediation Therapy in Chronic Schizophrenia. In B. Prasad (Ed.), *Chronic Mental Illness and the Changing Scope of Intervention Strategies, Diagnosis, and Treatment* (pp. 292–307). Hershey, PA: IGI Global. doi:10.4018/978-1-5225-0519-8.ch016

Hashim, A. H., Kaur, M., Bahar, N., & Ismail, W. S. (2016). Mental Health Issues among Family Members of Children with Mental Disability. In R. Gopalan (Ed.), *Handbook of Research on Diagnosing, Treating, and Managing Intellectual Disabilities* (pp. 54–81). Hershey, PA: IGI Global. doi:10.4018/978-1-5225-0089-6.ch004

Hazarika, M., & Choudhury, S. (2016). Attitude towards People with Intellectual Disabilities (PWID). In R. Gopalan (Ed.), *Handbook of Research on Diagnosing, Treating, and Managing Intellectual Disabilities* (pp. 237–261). Hershey, PA: IGI Global. doi:10.4018/978-1-5225-0089-6.ch013

Heins, S., Heins, G., & Dick-Muehlke, C. (2015). Steve's Story: Living with Mild Cognitive Impairment. In C. Dick-Muehlke, R. Li, & M. Orleans (Eds.), *Psychosocial Studies of the Individual's Changing Perspectives in Alzheimer's Disease* (pp. 33–60). Hershey, PA: IGI Global. doi:10.4018/978-1-4666-8478-2.ch002

Ho, W. T., & Fong, B. Y. (2018). Public-Private Partnership in Health and Long-Term Care: The Hong Kong Experience. In B. Fong, A. Ng, & P. Yuen (Eds.), *Sustainable Health and Long-Term Care Solutions for an Aging Population* (pp. 103–124). Hershey, PA: IGI Global. doi:10.4018/978-1-5225-2633-9.ch006

Hume, C., Hume, M., & Johnston, P. (2016). Creating Awareness and Practice: The ARCC@T Framework for Knowledge Management in Aged Care Services. *International Journal of Reliable and Quality E-Healthcare*, *5*(4), 1–14. doi:10.4018/IJRQEH.2016100101

Jagota, A., Jannu, N., & Boro, S. (2018). The Interplay of Biological and Socio Environmental Factors in Aging and Disorders in Women. In R. Pande & T. van der Weide (Eds.), *Handbook of Research on Multicultural Perspectives on Gender and Aging* (pp. 106–115). Hershey, PA: IGI Global. doi:10.4018/978-1-5225-4772-3.ch008

Jha, S., Khanna, A., & Khanna, P. (2017). Advanced Intervention Strategies for Suicide in Patients with Chronic Mental Illness. In B. Prasad (Ed.), *Chronic Mental Illness and the Changing Scope of Intervention Strategies, Diagnosis, and Treatment* (pp. 271–291). Hershey, PA: IGI Global. doi:10.4018/978-1-5225-0519-8.ch015

Kaushik, P., & Singh, T. B. (2017). Predictors of Expressed Emotion, Caregiver's Burden, and Quality of Life in Chronic Mental Illness. In B. Prasad (Ed.), *Chronic Mental Illness and the Changing Scope of Intervention Strategies, Diagnosis, and Treatment* (pp. 143–163). Hershey, PA: IGI Global. doi:10.4018/978-1-5225-0519-8.ch008

Khan, A. M., & Lawo, M. (2015). Recognizing Physical Activities using Wearable Devices. In P. Bamidis, I. Tarnanas, L. Hadjileontiadis, & M. Tsolaki (Eds.), *Handbook of Research on Innovations in the Diagnosis and Treatment of Dementia* (pp. 362–381). Hershey, PA: IGI Global. doi:10.4018/978-1-4666-8234-4.ch019

Kimaro, L. R. (2018). Gender and Elderly Care in Africa: A Challenge to Religious Institutions. In R. Pande & T. van der Weide (Eds.), *Handbook of Research on Multicultural Perspectives on Gender and Aging* (pp. 254–277). Hershey, PA: IGI Global. doi:10.4018/978-1-5225-4772-3.ch019

Kimotho, S. G. (2018). Understanding the Nature of Stigma Communication Associated With Mental Illness in Africa: A Focus on Cultural Beliefs and Stereotypes. In B. Canfield & H. Cunningham (Eds.), *Deconstructing Stigma in Mental Health* (pp. 20–41). Hershey, PA: IGI Global. doi:10.4018/978-1-5225-3808-0.ch002

Kram-Fernandez, D. (2018). Barriers to Practitioners' Endorsement of a Recovery Perspective: Considering Attitudes Through a Schema Lens. In B. Canfield & H. Cunningham (Eds.), *Deconstructing Stigma in Mental Health* (pp. 108–132). Hershey, PA: IGI Global. doi:10.4018/978-1-5225-3808-0.ch005

Kukreti, P., Khanna, P., & Khanna, A. (2017). Chronic Mental Illnesses and Homelessness. In B. Prasad (Ed.), *Chronic Mental Illness and the Changing Scope of Intervention Strategies, Diagnosis, and Treatment* (pp. 1–20). Hershey, PA: IGI Global. doi:10.4018/978-1-5225-0519-8.ch001

Lau, T., & Chan, K. (2018). Contributions of Volunteers in Long-Term Care in Hong Kong. In B. Fong, A. Ng, & P. Yuen (Eds.), *Sustainable Health and Long-Term Care Solutions for an Aging Population* (pp. 216–236). Hershey, PA: IGI Global. doi:10.4018/978-1-5225-2633-9.ch012

Law, V. T., & Ng, C. W. (2018). Corporate Social Responsibility of Long-Term Care Service Enterprises. In B. Fong, A. Ng, & P. Yuen (Eds.), *Sustainable Health and Long-Term Care Solutions for an Aging Population* (pp. 203–215). Hershey, PA: IGI Global. doi:10.4018/978-1-5225-2633-9.ch011

Lee, S. H. (2018). Rice Plus and Family Solidarity: Rural Cambodian Widows' Economic Coping Practices. In R. Pande & T. van der Weide (Eds.), *Handbook of Research on Multicultural Perspectives on Gender and Aging* (pp. 278–294). Hershey, PA: IGI Global. doi:10.4018/978-1-5225-4772-3.ch020

Leung, E., Chau, C. W., Lee, A., Chen, Y. F., & Lee, D. T. (2018). Integrated Care as a Strategic Solution for Active Aging in the Community: Tools and Models. In B. Fong, A. Ng, & P. Yuen (Eds.), *Sustainable Health and Long-Term Care Solutions for an Aging Population* (pp. 145–160). Hershey, PA: IGI Global. doi:10.4018/978-1-5225-2633-9.ch008

Lewy, H. (2015). Integrated Care: Technologies for Diagnosis and Treatment. In P. Bamidis, I. Tarnanas, L. Hadjileontiadis, & M. Tsolaki (Eds.), *Handbook of Research on Innovations in the Diagnosis and Treatment of Dementia* (pp. 163–174). Hershey, PA: IGI Global. doi:10.4018/978-1-4666-8234-4.ch009

Liu, K. Y., Wong, B. H., Chu, M., & Leung, W. Y. (2018). The Continuum of Care: A Case Study of a Senior Service Centre for Geriatric Care in Toronto, Canada. In B. Fong, A. Ng, & P. Yuen (Eds.), *Sustainable Health and Long-Term Care Solutions for an Aging Population* (pp. 71–90). Hershey, PA: IGI Global. doi:10.4018/978-1-5225-2633-9.ch004

Lo, M. F., & Ng, P. M. (2018). Knowledge Management for Health Care and Long-Term Care in the Technology-Organization-Environment Context. In B. Fong, A. Ng, & P. Yuen (Eds.), *Sustainable Health and Long-Term Care Solutions for an Aging Population* (pp. 161–186). Hershey, PA: IGI Global. doi:10.4018/978-1-5225-2633-9.ch009

Lu, Y. Y., & Austrom, M. G. (2015). Disease Awareness, Cognitive Decline, and Communication in Persons with Mild Cognitive Impairment and Caregivers. In C. Dick-Muehlke, R. Li, & M. Orleans (Eds.), *Psychosocial Studies of the Individual's Changing Perspectives in Alzheimer's Disease* (pp. 254–270). Hershey, PA: IGI Global. doi:10.4018/978-1-4666-8478-2.ch011

Luk, C. Y. (2018). Moving Towards Universal Health Coverage: Challenges for the Present and Future in China. In B. Fong, A. Ng, & P. Yuen (Eds.), *Sustainable Health and Long-Term Care Solutions for an Aging Population* (pp. 19–45). Hershey, PA: IGI Global. doi:10.4018/978-1-5225-2633-9.ch002

Lutwama-Rukundo, E., Kabonesa, C., & Nsibirano, R. (2018). That's My Space: Ageing, Gender, and Survival in Ugandan Theatre. In R. Pande & T. van der Weide (Eds.), *Handbook of Research on Multicultural Perspectives on Gender and Aging* (pp. 159–176). Hershey, PA: IGI Global. doi:10.4018/978-1-5225-4772-3.ch012

M., K., & Boominathan, P. (2016). Assessment and Management of Communication Skills in Individuals with Intellectual Disability: Perspectives in the 21st Century. In R. Gopalan (Ed.), *Handbook of Research on Diagnosing, Treating, and Managing Intellectual Disabilities* (pp. 156-185). Hershey, PA: IGI Global. doi:10.4018/978-1-5225-0089-6.ch009

MacKinlay, E., & Trevitt, C. (2015). Spiritual Factors in the Experience of Alzheimer's Disease and Other Dementias. In C. Dick-Muehlke, R. Li, & M. Orleans (Eds.), *Psychosocial Studies of the Individual's Changing Perspectives in Alzheimer's Disease* (pp. 230–253). Hershey, PA: IGI Global. doi:10.4018/978-1-4666-8478-2.ch010

Mahato, A., & Halder, S. (2017). Disability in Schizophrenia: The Psychosocial and Neurocognitive Perspective. In B. Prasad (Ed.), *Chronic Mental Illness and the Changing Scope of Intervention Strategies, Diagnosis, and Treatment* (pp. 188–202). Hershey, PA: IGI Global. doi:10.4018/978-1-5225-0519-8.ch010

Mitzner, T. L., & Dijkstra, K. (2016). Evaluating User Centered Design of E-Health for Older Adults: Using Subjective Methods. *International Journal of Computers in Clinical Practice, 1*(2), 24–50. doi:10.4018/IJCCP.2016070102

Morhardt, D., & Spira, M. (2015). Cognitive Decline and the Changing Self in Relationship. In C. Dick-Muehlke, R. Li, & M. Orleans (Eds.), *Psychosocial Studies of the Individual's Changing Perspectives in Alzheimer's Disease* (pp. 61–75). Hershey, PA: IGI Global. doi:10.4018/978-1-4666-8478-2.ch003

Mukherjee, S. (2018). Dementia: A Capability Deprivation for Elderly Women in India. In R. Pande & T. van der Weide (Eds.), *Handbook of Research on Multicultural Perspectives on Gender and Aging* (pp. 53–76). Hershey, PA: IGI Global. doi:10.4018/978-1-5225-4772-3.ch005

Nautiyal, A., & Bhatt, G. (2018). Socio-Psychological Complexities of Aging in Hill Areas of Upper Kedar Valley of Indian Mid-Central Himalayas. In R. Pande & T. van der Weide (Eds.), *Handbook of Research on Multicultural Perspectives on Gender and Aging* (pp. 217–230). Hershey, PA: IGI Global. doi:10.4018/978-1-5225-4772-3.ch016

Navarro, A. B., Díaz-Orueta, U., Martín-Niño, L., & Sánchez-Sánchez, M. E. (2015). Art, Drawing Task Processes, and Identity Awareness: A Case Study on the Retro-Genesis Phenomenon as an Indicator of the Progress of Dementia. In C. Dick-Muehlke, R. Li, & M. Orleans (Eds.), *Psychosocial Studies of the Individual's Changing Perspectives in Alzheimer's Disease* (pp. 208–228). Hershey, PA: IGI Global. doi:10.4018/978-1-4666-8478-2.ch009

Ng, A. W., Leung, T. C., & Ho, J. C. (2018). Development of Accreditation Approach of Elderly Care Service Providers: Experience from East and West. In B. Fong, A. Ng, & P. Yuen (Eds.), *Sustainable Health and Long-Term Care Solutions for an Aging Population* (pp. 126–144). Hershey, PA: IGI Global. doi:10.4018/978-1-5225-2633-9.ch007

Panda, P. K. (2018). Sustainable Development Plan for Aging World Population: Challenges and Way Forward. In R. Pande & T. van der Weide (Eds.), *Handbook of Research on Multicultural Perspectives on Gender and Aging* (pp. 26–36). Hershey, PA: IGI Global. doi:10.4018/978-1-5225-4772-3.ch003

Pande, R. (2018). The Forgotten Widows of Vrindavan in India. In R. Pande & T. van der Weide (Eds.), *Handbook of Research on Multicultural Perspectives on Gender and Aging* (pp. 200–216). Hershey, PA: IGI Global. doi:10.4018/978-1-5225-4772-3.ch015

Pandey, J. M., & Mishra, P. (2016). Intellectual Disability: An Awareness towards Intervention. In R. Gopalan (Ed.), *Handbook of Research on Diagnosing, Treating, and Managing Intellectual Disabilities* (pp. 220–236). Hershey, PA: IGI Global. doi:10.4018/978-1-5225-0089-6.ch012

Pandey, J. M., Mishra, P., Garg, S., & Mshra, B. P. (2017). Chronic Mental Illness and Dumping Patients: A Concern towards Management. In B. Prasad (Ed.), *Chronic Mental Illness and the Changing Scope of Intervention Strategies, Diagnosis, and Treatment* (pp. 40–57). Hershey, PA: IGI Global. doi:10.4018/978-1-5225-0519-8.ch003

Park, L. Q., & Busson, B. (2015). The Impact of Decline on Everyday Life in Alzheimer's Disease. In C. Dick-Muehlke, R. Li, & M. Orleans (Eds.), *Psychosocial Studies of the Individual's Changing Perspectives in Alzheimer's Disease* (pp. 327–338). Hershey, PA: IGI Global. doi:10.4018/978-1-4666-8478-2.ch014

Parmar, S. (2018). Women, Ageism, and Sexism: Changing Paradigms. In R. Pande & T. van der Weide (Eds.), *Handbook of Research on Multicultural Perspectives on Gender and Aging* (pp. 190–198). Hershey, PA: IGI Global. doi:10.4018/978-1-5225-4772-3.ch014

Petridis, S., Giannakopoulos, T., & Perantonis, S. (2015). Unobtrusive Low-Cost Physiological Monitoring Using Visual Information. In P. Bamidis, I. Tarnanas, L. Hadjileontiadis, & M. Tsolaki (Eds.), *Handbook of Research on Innovations in the Diagnosis and Treatment of Dementia* (pp. 306–316). Hershey, PA: IGI Global. doi:10.4018/978-1-4666-8234-4.ch016

Power, G. A. (2015). Changing Perception in Alzheimer's: An Experiential View. In C. Dick-Muehlke, R. Li, & M. Orleans (Eds.), *Psychosocial Studies of the Individual's Changing Perspectives in Alzheimer's Disease* (pp. 271–300). Hershey, PA: IGI Global. doi:10.4018/978-1-4666-8478-2.ch012

Prusty, B. (2016). The Stress and Adjustment in the Family of Intellectually Disabled Children. In R. Gopalan (Ed.), *Handbook of Research on Diagnosing, Treating, and Managing Intellectual Disabilities* (pp. 82–108). Hershey, PA: IGI Global. doi:10.4018/978-1-5225-0089-6.ch005

R., A., Prasad, B. V., & Kosgi, S. (2017). Psychosocial Intervention Strategies for Patients with Schizophrenia: In Chronic Mental Illness. In B. Prasad (Ed.), *Chronic Mental Illness and the Changing Scope of Intervention Strategies, Diagnosis, and Treatment* (pp. 58-75). Hershey, PA: IGI Global. doi:10.4018/978-1-5225-0519-8.ch004

Rajesh, M. N. (2018). Getting Old in Little Lhasa: Experiences of Aging in Dharamsala. In R. Pande & T. van der Weide (Eds.), *Handbook of Research on Multicultural Perspectives on Gender and Aging* (pp. 177–189). Hershey, PA: IGI Global. doi:10.4018/978-1-5225-4772-3.ch013

Rodil, K., Nielsen, E. B., & Nielsen, J. B. (2018). Sharing Memories: Co-Designing Assistive Technology with Aphasic Adults and Support Staff. *International Journal of Sociotechnology and Knowledge Development*, *10*(1), 21–36. doi:10.4018/IJSKD.2018010102

Romanopoulou, E. D., Zilidou, V. I., & Antoniou, P. E. (2015). Spinning off Gerotechnology Business Activities: The LLM Care Best Practice Paradigm. In P. Bamidis, I. Tarnanas, L. Hadjileontiadis, & M. Tsolaki (Eds.), *Handbook of Research on Innovations in the Diagnosis and Treatment of Dementia* (pp. 426–436). Hershey, PA: IGI Global. doi:10.4018/978-1-4666-8234-4.ch023

S., I. R., & S., S. (2018). Impact of Widowhood and Disability Among Elderly. In R. Pande, & T. van der Weide (Eds.), *Handbook of Research on Multicultural Perspectives on Gender and Aging* (pp. 38-52). Hershey, PA: IGI Global. doi:10.4018/978-1-5225-4772-3.ch004

Sahu, R. (2018). Demographic Transition in India: Issues and Concerns. In R. Pande & T. van der Weide (Eds.), *Handbook of Research on Multicultural Perspectives on Gender and Aging* (pp. 117–125). Hershey, PA: IGI Global. doi:10.4018/978-1-5225-4772-3.ch009

Santhosh, K. R. (2016). Stress and Resilience in Parents of Intellectually Disabled Children. In R. Gopalan (Ed.), *Handbook of Research on Diagnosing, Treating, and Managing Intellectual Disabilities* (pp. 109–117). Hershey, PA: IGI Global. doi:10.4018/978-1-5225-0089-6.ch006

Schmeida, M., & McNeal, R. (2016). Consulting Online Healthcare Information: E-Caregivers as Knowledgeable Decision Makers. *International Journal of Computers in Clinical Practice*, *1*(1), 42–52. doi:10.4018/IJCCP.2016010104

Schmeida, M., & McNeal, R. S. (2018). Long-Term Care Spending Relevant to U.S. Medicaid Expansion: Medicaid Long-Term Care Spending. In B. Fong, A. Ng, & P. Yuen (Eds.), *Sustainable Health and Long-Term Care Solutions for an Aging Population* (pp. 46–70). Hershey, PA: IGI Global. doi:10.4018/978-1-5225-2633-9.ch003

Segkouli, S., Paliokas, I., Tsakiris, T., Votis, K., & Tzovaras, D. (2015). Enabling Accessibility Features in Enhanced VR Environments for Supporting Spatial Abilities and Social Interaction in Elderly and MCI Patients. In P. Bamidis, I. Tarnanas, L. Hadjileontiadis, & M. Tsolaki (Eds.), *Handbook of Research on Innovations in the Diagnosis and Treatment of Dementia* (pp. 147–162). Hershey, PA: IGI Global. doi:10.4018/978-1-4666-8234-4.ch008

Sernani, P., Claudi, A., & Dragoni, A. F. (2015). Combining Artificial Intelligence and NetMedicine for Ambient Assisted Living: A Distributed BDI-based Expert System. *International Journal of E-Health and Medical Communications*, *6*(4), 62–76. doi:10.4018/IJEHMC.2015100105

Sharma, R., & Lohan, A. (2016). Psychosocial Interventions for Individuals with Intellectual Disability. In R. Gopalan (Ed.), *Handbook of Research on Diagnosing, Treating, and Managing Intellectual Disabilities* (pp. 262–282). Hershey, PA: IGI Global. doi:10.4018/978-1-5225-0089-6.ch014

Sharon, D. (2015). The Sleep-Wake System and Alzheimer's Disease. In C. Dick-Muehlke, R. Li, & M. Orleans (Eds.), *Psychosocial Studies of the Individual's Changing Perspectives in Alzheimer's Disease* (pp. 339–365). Hershey, PA: IGI Global. doi:10.4018/978-1-4666-8478-2.ch015

Sidiropoulos, E. A., Zilidou, V. I., Karagianni, M. A., Ioannidis, L. I., Romanopoulou, E. D., Karagiozi, K. I., ... Bamidis, P. D. (2015). ICT Support to Those Providing Care to Elderly: Pilot Training Activities in Greece in the Realm of the DISCOVER Project. In P. Bamidis, I. Tarnanas, L. Hadjileontiadis, & M. Tsolaki (Eds.), *Handbook of Research on Innovations in the Diagnosis and Treatment of Dementia* (pp. 397–413). Hershey, PA: IGI Global. doi:10.4018/978-1-4666-8234-4.ch021

Sinha, P., Garg, A., Khanna, P., & Khanna, A. (2017). Management of Chronic Mental Illnesses and Substance Use Disorders. In B. Prasad (Ed.), *Chronic Mental Illness and the Changing Scope of Intervention Strategies, Diagnosis, and Treatment* (pp. 101–122). Hershey, PA: IGI Global. doi:10.4018/978-1-5225-0519-8.ch006

Soni, S. C. P., & Ahamed, P. C. (2017). Understanding and Management of Caregivers' Stress and Burden of Person with Obsessive Compulsive Disorder. In B. Prasad (Ed.), *Chronic Mental Illness and the Changing Scope of Intervention Strategies, Diagnosis, and Treatment* (pp. 124–142). Hershey, PA: IGI Global. doi:10.4018/978-1-5225-0519-8.ch007

Srivastav, D., & Singh, T. B. (2017). Comorbidity Issues and Treatment in Chronic Mental Illness. In B. Prasad (Ed.), *Chronic Mental Illness and the Changing Scope of Intervention Strategies, Diagnosis, and Treatment* (pp. 77–100). Hershey, PA: IGI Global. doi:10.4018/978-1-5225-0519-8.ch005

Styliadis, C., Kartsidis, P., & Paraskevopoulos, E. (2015). Neuroimaging Approaches for Elderly Studies. In P. Bamidis, I. Tarnanas, L. Hadjileontiadis, & M. Tsolaki (Eds.), *Handbook of Research on Innovations in the Diagnosis and Treatment of Dementia* (pp. 47–86). Hershey, PA: IGI Global. doi:10.4018/978-1-4666-8234-4.ch004

Svanström, R. (2015). Fragmented Existence: Living Alone with Dementia and a Manifest Care Need. In C. Dick-Muehlke, R. Li, & M. Orleans (Eds.), *Psychosocial Studies of the Individual's Changing Perspectives in Alzheimer's Disease* (pp. 302–326). Hershey, PA: IGI Global. doi:10.4018/978-1-4666-8478-2.ch013

Tarnanas, I., Tsolakis, A., & Tsolaki, M. (2015). Cognitive Exercising for Patients with MCI Using Serious Games: Design of a Pilot Study. In P. Bamidis, I. Tarnanas, L. Hadjileontiadis, & M. Tsolaki (Eds.), *Handbook of Research on Innovations in the Diagnosis and Treatment of Dementia* (pp. 88–117). Hershey, PA: IGI Global. doi:10.4018/978-1-4666-8234-4.ch005

Tavaragi, M. S. (2017). Chronic Mental Illness in Prisons: Global Scenario. In B. Prasad (Ed.), *Chronic Mental Illness and the Changing Scope of Intervention Strategies, Diagnosis, and Treatment* (pp. 203–224). Hershey, PA: IGI Global. doi:10.4018/978-1-5225-0519-8.ch011

Tavaragi, M. S., & C., S. (2017). Global Burden of Mental Disorders: Quality of Care and Unmet Needs for Treatment of Chronic Mental Illness. In B. Prasad (Ed.), *Chronic Mental Illness and the Changing Scope of Intervention Strategies, Diagnosis, and Treatment* (pp. 164-186). Hershey, PA: IGI Global. doi:10.4018/978-1-5225-0519-8.ch009

Toms, G., Lawrence, C., & Clare, L. (2015). Awareness, Self, and the Experience of Dementia: Foundations of a Psychologically Minded Approach. In C. Dick-Muehlke, R. Li, & M. Orleans (Eds.), *Psychosocial Studies of the Individual's Changing Perspectives in Alzheimer's Disease* (pp. 132–158). Hershey, PA: IGI Global. doi:10.4018/978-1-4666-8478-2.ch006

Tong, K., & Fong, K. N. (2018). Community-Based Rehabilitation in Hong Kong: Opportunities and Challenges. In B. Fong, A. Ng, & P. Yuen (Eds.), *Sustainable Health and Long-Term Care Solutions for an Aging Population* (pp. 294–319). Hershey, PA: IGI Global. doi:10.4018/978-1-5225-2633-9.ch016

Tran, B. (2018). Understanding and Addressing the Stigma in Mental Health Within the Asian and Asian-American Culture. In B. Canfield & H. Cunningham (Eds.), *Deconstructing Stigma in Mental Health* (pp. 70–107). Hershey, PA: IGI Global. doi:10.4018/978-1-5225-3808-0.ch004

Tripathi, M. A., & Sridevi, G. (2017). Psychotherapeutic Interventions in Emotional and Behavioural Problems with Adolescents. In B. Prasad (Ed.), *Chronic Mental Illness and the Changing Scope of Intervention Strategies, Diagnosis, and Treatment* (pp. 321–333). Hershey, PA: IGI Global. doi:10.4018/978-1-5225-0519-8.ch018

Tsang, K. T., & Ip, C. F. (2018). SSLD and Senior Service: A Comprehensive Model for Practice. In B. Fong, A. Ng, & P. Yuen (Eds.), *Sustainable Health and Long-Term Care Solutions for an Aging Population* (pp. 238–258). Hershey, PA: IGI Global. doi:10.4018/978-1-5225-2633-9.ch013

Tsolaki, A. (2015). "Personal Training": Can Genes Guide Us? In P. Bamidis, I. Tarnanas, L. Hadjileontiadis, & M. Tsolaki (Eds.), *Handbook of Research on Innovations in the Diagnosis and Treatment of Dementia* (pp. 18–36). Hershey, PA: IGI Global. doi:10.4018/978-1-4666-8234-4.ch002

Uprety, S., & Ghimire, R. (2018). Media, Social Media, and the Securitization of Mental Health Problems in Nepal: Yama Buddha's Case Study. In B. Canfield & H. Cunningham (Eds.), *Deconstructing Stigma in Mental Health* (pp. 42–69). Hershey, PA: IGI Global. doi:10.4018/978-1-5225-3808-0.ch003

van der Weide, T. (2018). Self-Esteem During the Ageing Process. In R. Pande & T. van der Weide (Eds.), *Handbook of Research on Multicultural Perspectives on Gender and Aging* (pp. 88–105). Hershey, PA: IGI Global. doi:10.4018/978-1-5225-4772-3.ch007

Verma, S. (2018). Feminization of Old Age and Experiences of Subalternity: The Socio-Cultural Dynamics of Inclusion – Exclusion in Urban India. In R. Pande & T. van der Weide (Eds.), *Handbook of Research on Multicultural Perspectives on Gender and Aging* (pp. 77–87). Hershey, PA: IGI Global. doi:10.4018/978-1-5225-4772-3.ch006

von Kutzleben, M., & Panke-Kochinke, B. (2015). Stable Self-Concepts and Flexible Coping Strategies of People with Dementia Attending Dementia Self-Help Groups in Germany: Results from the Qualitative Longitudinal SEIN Study. In C. Dick-Muehlke, R. Li, & M. Orleans (Eds.), *Psychosocial Studies of the Individual's Changing Perspectives in Alzheimer's Disease* (pp. 159–182). Hershey, PA: IGI Global. doi:10.4018/978-1-4666-8478-2.ch007

Vontas, A., Moumtzi, V., & Urwin, G. (2015). Spinning Off Business Activities for Care Giver Support: The DISCOVER Attempt. In P. Bamidis, I. Tarnanas, L. Hadjileontiadis, & M. Tsolaki (Eds.), *Handbook of Research on Innovations in the Diagnosis and Treatment of Dementia* (pp. 414–425). Hershey, PA: IGI Global. doi:10.4018/978-1-4666-8234-4.ch022

Vora, K. S. (2016). Family Members as Caregivers of Individuals with Intellectual Disabilities: Caregiving for Individuals with Intellectual Disabilities. In R. Gopalan (Ed.), *Handbook of Research on Diagnosing, Treating, and Managing Intellectual Disabilities* (pp. 118–138). Hershey, PA: IGI Global. doi:10.4018/978-1-5225-0089-6.ch007

Votis, K., Segkouli, S., Drosou, A., Tzovaras, D., & Tsolaki, M. (2015). An Ambient Intelligence System for the Monitoring, Empowerment, and Disease Evolution Prediction for Patients with Mild Cognitive Impairment. In P. Bamidis, I. Tarnanas, L. Hadjileontiadis, & M. Tsolaki (Eds.), *Handbook of Research on Innovations in the Diagnosis and Treatment of Dementia* (pp. 225–239). Hershey, PA: IGI Global. doi:10.4018/978-1-4666-8234-4.ch012

Wong, A. K., & Lo, M. F. (2018). Using Pervasive Computing for Sustainable Healthcare in an Aging Population. In B. Fong, A. Ng, & P. Yuen (Eds.), *Sustainable Health and Long-Term Care Solutions for an Aging Population* (pp. 187–202). Hershey, PA: IGI Global. doi:10.4018/978-1-5225-2633-9.ch010

Woo, R. K., Kwok, A. O., & Tse, D. M. (2018). Preferred Place of Care and Death Among the Terminally Ill: Asian Perspectives and Implications for Hong Kong. In B. Fong, A. Ng, & P. Yuen (Eds.), *Sustainable Health and Long-Term Care Solutions for an Aging Population* (pp. 277–293). Hershey, PA: IGI Global. doi:10.4018/978-1-5225-2633-9.ch015

Wright, M. F. (2016). School Bullying and Students with Intellectual Disabilities. In R. Gopalan (Ed.), *Handbook of Research on Diagnosing, Treating, and Managing Intellectual Disabilities* (pp. 33–53). Hershey, PA: IGI Global. doi:10.4018/978-1-5225-0089-6.ch003

Xenakidis, C. N., Hadjiantonis, A. M., & Milis, G. M. (2015). Assistive Technologies for People with Dementia. In P. Bamidis, I. Tarnanas, L. Hadjileontiadis, & M. Tsolaki (Eds.), *Handbook of Research on Innovations in the Diagnosis and Treatment of Dementia* (pp. 269–289). Hershey, PA: IGI Global. doi:10.4018/978-1-4666-8234-4.ch014

Yuen, P. P. (2018). The Economics of Long-Term Care: Key Concepts and Major Financing and Delivery Models. In B. Fong, A. Ng, & P. Yuen (Eds.), *Sustainable Health and Long-Term Care Solutions for an Aging Population* (pp. 1–18). Hershey, PA: IGI Global. doi:10.4018/978-1-5225-2633-9.ch001

Zygouris, S., & Tsolaki, M. (2015). New Technologies and Neuropsychological Evaluation of Older Adults: Issues and Challenges. In P. Bamidis, I. Tarnanas, L. Hadjileontiadis, & M. Tsolaki (Eds.), *Handbook of Research on Innovations in the Diagnosis and Treatment of Dementia* (pp. 1–17). Hershey, PA: IGI Global. doi:10.4018/978-1-4666-8234-4.ch001

About the Authors

Debra Gavin Ware obtained a Bachelor's degree in Political Science from Bradley University in Peoria, Illinois (1983). She completed her Master of Science degree in Non-Profit Management from Spertus College in Chicago, Illinois (2012). She completed her doctoral degree in Education specializing in Organizational Leadership from Argosy University in Chicago, Illinois (2016). She served as President of the Sigma Beta Delta honor society from 2012 to 2014. Dr. Gavin Ware is an Adjunct Professor at Argosy University teaching undergraduate and doctoral students. She serves as a dissertation coach, committee member and mentor for several doctoral students. She is an active member of the Toast Master's International organization. Her research interests include areas such as adult bullying, aging advocacy, factors affecting Informal Caregivers and non-profit leadership.

Tarnue Johnson obtained an MA degree in political economy from Middlesex University in London, UK (1992-94). Dr. Johnson completed a postgraduate certificate in adult education at the Institute of Education, University College London (1995-96). He spent a year doing postgraduate studies in educational research, policy and planning at the University of Manchester in Manchester, UK (1997-98). Dr. Johnson completed his Doctorate in Business Administration (DBA) at Argosy University/Chicago with concentration in management (2007-11). He also completed postdoctoral studies at Northwestern University in Chicago (2015). Dr. Johnson has authored and co-authored more than seven books---with several in the pipeline---in collaboration with leading American, African American and African scholars and intellectuals. He has also written and published several peer-reviewed articles in reputable journals. His research interests include globalization and business ethics, public policy and neuro organizational cognitive science. The author has also taught at various colleges and universities in Illinois and Iowa.

Index

S

T

V

W

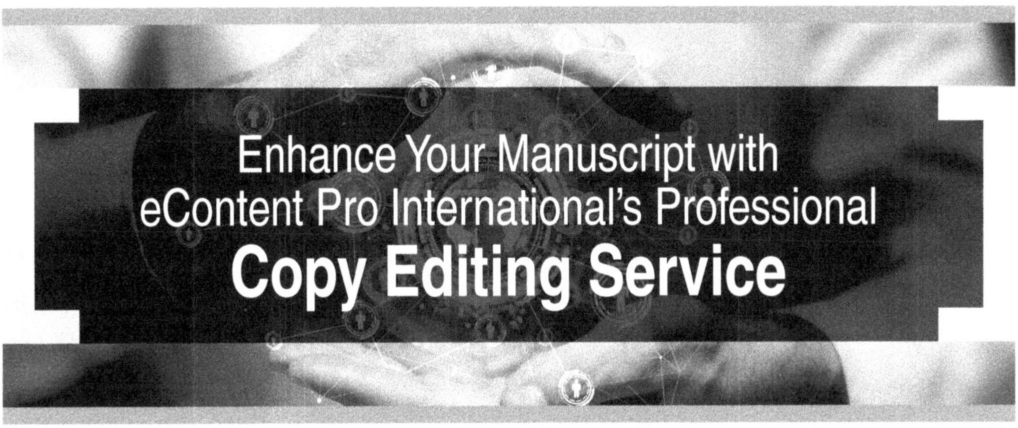
Enhance Your Manuscript with
eContent Pro International's Professional
Copy Editing Service

www.ingramcontent.com/pod-product-compliance
Lightning Source LLC
LaVergne TN
LVHW081330021026
849161LV00008BA/1831